T0281110

The Psychology of Neurogenic Communication Disorders

A Primer for Health Care Professionals

Dennis C. Tanner
Northern Arizona University

iUniverse, Inc.
New York   Bloomington

The Psychology of Neurogenic Communication Disorders:
A Primer for Health Care Professionals

iUniverse books may be ordered through booksellers or by contacting:

iUniverse
1663 Liberty Drive
Bloomington, IN 47403
www.iuniverse.com
1-800-Authors (1-800-288-4677)

Because of the dynamic nature of the Internet, any Web addresses or links contained in this book may have changed since publication and may no longer be valid. The views expressed in this work are solely those of the author and do not necessarily reflect the views of the publisher, and the publisher hereby disclaims any responsibility for them.

ISBN: 978-1-4401-8195-5 (pbk)

This book was previously published by: Pearson Education, Inc.

Printed in the United States of America

iUniverse rev. date: 10/22/09

CONTENTS

PART TWO   On Coping with Neurogenic
Communication Disorders:
Original Short Stories   89

FIGURES

TABLES

FOREWORD

The Psychology of Neurogenic Communication Disorders: A Primer for Health Care Professionals is an important book for people who will come in contact with patients suffering from neurogenic speech, language, and communication deficits. Textbooks and courses in this area too often stress only the anatomy and physiology of the mechanisms underlying neurogenic communication disorders and leave out important psychological considerations about the patient that health care professionals must deal with on a daily basis. This book bridges that important gap.

This book is important because it enters the realm of realism. Having worked in rehabilitation for several years and having taught neurology of communication disorders for over 10 years, I recognize the importance of considering the whole person. For many individuals the psychological sequelae following a neurological injury are at least as debilitating as the actual physical symptoms. This book treats those psychological factors with the necessary importance and explains them in a clear and comprehensive fashion.

It is true that the field of neurogenic communication disorders is based upon strong, scientifically "provable" models, i.e., the theory of localization. However, some researchers, authors, and clinicians have argued for the abstractness of human thought and contend that the brain and the psyche operate holistically, rather than as a collection of individual parts. I have heard many social scientists state that human beings are notoriously difficult to study with only one method of scientific inquiry. I interpret these wise warnings as indications that we just don't know all there is to know about the neurology and psychology of communication disorders. If we knew all there was to know about human behaviors, modern brain imaging techniques would be the sole tool required to identify the symptoms, strengths, and weaknesses of our patients with neurogenically based communication disorders. Obviously much more than that is needed. I have personally witnessed patients perform a given task that clinical tools of the trade indicated were physically impossible. The opposite is also true. Why do some patients function quite well with a condition that would be debilitating to another? It is obvious to many that a multitude of factors contribute to the make-up of complex human behavior. This text provides excellent information for the professional working with patients who have neurologically based communication disorders, and it adds important information about psychological factors as well. A true step forward in patient care.

This book is unique in that it offers more than a sound review of neurogenic communication disorders. It also offers a more humanistic approach for students and professionals who are just becoming familiar with human communication disorders. In my years of teaching about neurological communication disorders, students often commented on the importance of practical experiences and how the "stories" that I told in class pulled together the theoretical information I was lecturing on. Dennis Tanner's book follows this pattern by actually providing the true-life stories and clinical vignettes that enhance learning. Part II of this textbook is a rare and valuable humanistic view of neurogenic communication disorders. This section is invaluable for the true understanding it provides of the complexities involved with neurogenic communication disorders. The concept of looking at the whole person and describing all of their symptoms, not just the ones that can be charted on a brain map, is a valuable addition to the current literature in this area.

It is certainly the goal of educators to reach their students. I believe that Dennis Tanner's text will effectively reach students inclined to learn about the psychology of communication disorders. This text views the person as a whole. Neurological communication disorders affect more than the brain, they affect the person's entire world, including their human psyche and social participation. Duchan (2000) has recently stated, "the trends in assessment (of communication disorders) broaden the view of communication to include everyday social participation" (p. 191). The trend is obviously starting and picking up momentum. The functionality of communication is being viewed as an important aspect in the assessment and rehabilitation of communication disorders. This functional approach has been called for, and it is gaining even more momentum through descriptive techniques in aphasiology and other communication disorders (see Damico, Oelschlaeger, and Simmons-Mackie, 1999; Tetnowski and Damico, 2001). If we are going to study human communication disorders in a meaningful fashion, we must understand the exactness provided by objective, scientific inquiry of neurology from a "localizationist" point of view, but we also must be aware of how the psyche of the human species affects their behavior. Dennis Tanner's book is a step in this direction.

Psychological issues can have an impact on otherwise clear, understandable diagnoses. If we are to treat the whole person, we must understand the importance of psychological factors surrounding neurogenic communication disorders. This book is a rare and important document that enters this realm. Now that I have read the manuscript, I could not legitimize teaching a course in human, neurological communication disorders without including a section that introduces the importance of the psychology involved with neurogenic insult. Thank you, Dennis Tanner, for putting this into book into press.

Finally, I would like to leave a note for the reader. We often have goals for our actions. Your goal for reading this book or studying in this area may be that you want to enter a profession that comes in contact with neurogenic communication disorders; or your goal may be to find out more information about a family member with a neurogenic communication disorder; or your goal may be that your job requires a better understanding of neurogenic communication disorders. Whatever your goal is, I hope that you meet your goals, but I also urge you to enjoy the process along the way. Dennis Tanner has made this possible through his wonderfully clear and insightful view of neurogenic communication disorders. Enjoy your journey!

John A. Tetnowski, Ph.D., CCC-SLP
University of Louisiana at Lafayette
Lafayette, Louisiana

PREFACE

This book is about the psychology of neurogenic communication disorders. It is written about patients who have aphasia, apraxia of speech, and/or the dysarthrias. It is intended as a guide to understanding the significant psychological adjustments many patients must undergo.

This book is written for health care professionals. Whether the reader is a student, physician, neuropsychologist, counselor, nurse, occupational or physical therapist, or speech-language pathologist, the information found herein is intended to provide insight into the psychological status of the patient. Current and meaningful information is provided to assist in evaluating and treating patients with neurogenic communication disorders.

This is a nontraditional book. There are short stories, clinical vignettes, and case studies to help the reader appreciate and understand the psychological transitions many patients experience. Some are actual clinical cases or composites of several patients, and others are fictional accounts addressing communication disorders and likely psychological reactions to them. The goal is to present the material in an interesting way, one that personally involves the reader.

The information provided herein is a result of the author's clinical experience, research, and study in the psychology of neurogenic communication disorders. Every effort has been made to use terminology easily understood by professionals from a variety of disciplines. When technical terms are used, they are defined or described. Hopefully, this book provides a foundation for understanding the many psychological changes experienced by people with neurogenic communication disorders.

Dennis C. Tanner, Ph.D.
Flagstaff, Arizona

ACKNOWLEDGMENTS

Several people helped me immensely during the writing of this book. First, thanks to Drs. James Blagg, William Culbertson, and Wayne Secord for their interest in the topic and much appreciated encouragement. Second, thanks also to Stacey Bolar, Cindy Dambach, Valerie Haunschild, Deseré Henderson, and Heather Lafferty for their help with research, illustrations, tables, and typing. Third, to Viktoria Kristiansson, thank you for appreciating the importance of the psychological issues in patients with neurogenic communication disorders and for your help and counsel in conceptualizing this book. Finally, thanks to reviewers: Carole T. Ferrand, Hofstra University; Celia R. Hooper, University of North Carolina; and Robert J. Logan, University of Central Arkansas, for their suggestions on how to improve the content, and to the professionals at Allyn & Bacon for their support and know-how in turning ideas into a book.

ABOUT THE AUTHOR

Dennis C. Tanner received a Doctor of Philosophy degree in Audiology and Speech Sciences, with a minor in Psychiatry from Michigan State University in 1976. He has published or presented over ninety books, tests, articles, and papers, many on neurogenic communication disorders.

During his career, Dr. Tanner has studied extensively psychology and quality of life issues of patients with aphasia, apraxia of speech, and the dysarthrias. He, with psychiatrist Dr. Dean Gerstenberger, has explored several dimensions of psychological reactions in aphasic patients, the results of which have been published in the international, interdisciplinary journal *Aphasiology*. Other published papers about the psychology of neurogenic communication disorders have addressed loss, grief, chronic depression, nursing considerations, culture care issues, and disorientation in brain injured persons. He has also copresented two minicourses on the psychology of aphasia and related disorders at conventions of the American Speech-Language-Hearing Association. Books and tests addressing the psychology of neurogenic communication disorders include *Aphasia: Coping with Unwanted Change, An Introduction to the Psychology of Aphasia, The Family Guide to Surviving Stroke and Communication Disorders, The Caregiver-Administered Communication Inventory* and the *Quick Assessment Series for Neurogenic Communication Disorders* (with Dr. William Culbertson). He is also the author of the *Aphasic Patient's Bill of Rights*.

Dr. Tanner and his wife, Jody, are owners of *Tanner Rehabilitation Services, Inc.*, which has provided speech and hearing services to individuals, hospitals, nursing homes, home health organizations, and government agencies in northern Arizona for twenty-five years. He also serves as an expert witness in legal cases involving patients with communication and swallowing disorders. Dr. Tanner is currently Professor of Communication Sciences and Disorders at Northern Arizona University in Flagstaff, Arizona and is one of two recipients of the Association of Schools of Allied Health Professions' "Outstanding Educator Award" for 2001–2002.

PART I

An Eclectic Approach to the Psychology of Neurogenic Communication Disorders

> *To say a clinician must be aware of psychological problems in aphasia is to say he must be aware that he is dealing with people. Sometimes we are so intimidated by labels, such as emotional lability, catastrophic reactions, anxiety, depression, euphoria, etc., that we forget this first principle. We talk trade jargon with glibness that betrays our dearth of insights. We talk as though aphasic patients were different from everyone else, and we had to have a different set of rules for dealing with them.*
>
> —Schuell, Jenkins, and Jimenez-Pabon, 1964, p. 315

1 Historical Perspectives on the Psychology of Neurogenic Communication Disorders

"If I have seen farther it is by standing on the shoulders of giants."

—Issac Newton

Introduction

Neurogenic communication disorders—aphasia, apraxia of speech, and the dysarthrias—can be psychologically devastating. These disorders, often accompanied by significant limitations on many activities of daily living, can lay waste to the ability to communicate. Not only can these communication disorders profoundly alter the lives of those afflicted by them, they can drive a wedge between the patient and his or her loved ones. This happens at a time when the patient needs to reach out for support and understanding. Psychologically, neurogenic communication disorders are double-edged swords. They are often caused by serious chronic medical conditions encompassing many adjustment challenges, and they can sever communication between the patient and those who can and want to help. Neurogenic communication disorders can cut a wide swath in the quality of life of those people afflicted by them.

The purpose of this book is to review the major neurogenic communication disorders and to provide a model by which clinicians from many disciplines can understand the psychological aspects of them. Prior to exploring the psychology of these communication disorders, a general review of their speech and language clinical manifestations is offered. While comprehensive, this review is not intended to serve as a substitute for texts on neurogenic communication disorders. It is designed to give readers from a variety of disciplines and educational levels a basic understanding of these complicated disorders.

It is proposed that psychological changes in patients with aphasia and related disorders can result from 1) organic and biochemical alterations occurring as a direct result of the brain damage, 2) activation and/or breakdown of premorbid coping styles and psychological defenses, and 3) reaction to loss. Although this separation is made for descriptive purposes, it should be noted that, on a practical level, the multiple determinants of psychological reactions seen in neurogenic communication disorders cannot be meaningfully separated.

Over the past three or four decades, two schools of thought have evolved in the world of psychology and psychiatry. One school is made up of people who believe that anxiety, depression, hostility, attention deficits, psychosis, and other psychological reactions are the result of either brain chemicals gone awry or brain injury. In this book, these clinicians, researchers, and theorists are referred to as *localizationists*, and a review of their accomplishments is provided. These clinicians, researchers, and theorists focus on pinpointing a part of the brain responsible for this, that or the other psychological phenomenon. They engage in brain mapping studies and explore the brain rather than the "mind." The other school, *nonlocalizationists*, consists of clinicians, researchers, and theorists who look at the brain and psychological functioning holistically. They believe that anxiety, depression, hostility, attention deficits, psychosis, and other psychological reactions should be viewed not only as a result of brain aberrations, but also seen through the processes of the mind. In the first school, psychologically and emotionally disordered individuals are victims of deficient or imbalanced brain chemistry. In the second school, they have self-determination and are capable of improving their lives through environmental changes, counseling, introspection, changes in cognitive processing, and improved family support. Some authorities refer to these schools as the *medical* and *social* models. There is value in both schools, of course, but they have important philosophical differences.

A good example of this dichotomy surrounds clinical depression. For the strict localizationist, a depressed person has a chemical imbalance, and in the case of stroke and aphasia, it is the result of damage to specific areas of the brain. To resolve the depression, antidepressants are prescribed to counter the chemical imbalance. In most cases, the person's depression lifts, but he or she may still be in unsatisfying relationships, confined to a cold and nonstimulating institution, jobless, grieving over the loss of speech and language, separated from loved ones, and/or engaging in psychological patterns of thought and adjustment that are unproductive or even self-defeating. With the administration of antidepressants the depression lifts, but the underlying social and psychological aspects of the illness persist.

Certainly, some people are depressed simply because of an imbalance of brain chemicals, and this course of treatment is appropriate and warranted. In many patients with aphasia, apraxia of speech, and the dysarthrias, however, depression is much more than a chemical imbalance, and the quick and cheap fix of only antidepressant medication therapy is shortsighted, negligent and dehumanizing. In the current health-care economic climate, this approach is emphasized even though it avoids confronting the real problems associated with or underlying the depression. This philosophy for treating psychological problems in patients with neurogenic communication disorders is shortsighted and superficial.

The majority of current research into the psychology of neurogenic communication disorders involves localization issues. The goal is to identify sites in the brain that, when damaged, cause denial, anxiety, depression, euphoria, and a host of other psychological reactions. However, it should be remembered that localizing the site where certain emotional reactions occur, or identifying a chemical deficiency in the brain, is not comprehensive scientific exploration into the psychology of these disorders. Simply pointing to a chemical deficiency or a damaged tract of axons is not the same as exploring the myriad of causes, symptoms, and treatment options.

Part I, the theoretical aspect of this book, provides a treatise on the psychology of neurogenic communication disorders. It has major implications for understanding and treating patients with aphasia, apraxia of speech, and the dysarthrias. The clinical vignettes, case examples, and Part II: Short Stories are included for pedagogical purposes. They are provided primarily for students and beginning professionals who may not have experience with these patients. They are designed to add interest and to help explain the information.

To Localize or Not to Localize

The thrust of early research into neurogenic communication disorders was to locate areas of the brain that were responsible for specific speech and language functions. Sies (1974) and Benson and Ardila (1996) have provided detailed histories of the speech and language localization movement. This desire to localize functional speech and language areas of the brain, or *modules*, continues today. *Modules* are areas of the brain devoted to specific functions or processing activities (Owens, Metz, & Haas, 2000). Researchers use sophisticated brain scanning devices and attempt to pinpoint areas of the brain responsible for specific functions. A strict localizationist philosophy of brain functioning is difficult to support because no single part of the brain functions completely independent from the others. For example, although certain identifiable areas of the brain may be central to perceiving vowels and consonants, pin-pointing the mass of brain cells completely responsible, in every person, for interpreting a proverb or understanding the implications of a Robert Frost poem is absurd. And, of course, there is the monumental task of identifying neurochemical activities in the cells of the brain and projecting what happens in a particular person's mind. Given current technology and scientific advances, the brain-mind leap is insurmountably complex and compounded by extreme individual variation.

In the past, as today, not all teachers, researchers, and clinicians in neurogenic communication disorders rode the localization bandwagon. An early critic of the theories of localization was Henry Head. Head was critical particularly of researchers of the day who assumed that "pure" neurogenic speech and language disorders exist. Head believed it was unproductive to list speech and language functions or to create a diagram showing the areas of the brain responsible for all of them. Head recognized that the brain operates holistically (Sies, 1974, Benson & Ardila, 1996).

Over time, schools of thought regarding aphasia and related disorders were formed. Perhaps it is because of the complexity of these disorders that many present-day teachers, researchers, and clinicians adhere so rigidly to the doctrines of those philosophies about neurogenic communication disorders. Those early schools of thought, and many others, make basic assumptions about the cognitive and psychological makeup of patients with neurogenic communication disorders.

The *association* school of thought assumes that aphasic disorders are disturbances in labeling ideas, objects, or events (Benton, 1981). Adherents to this school think that the basic intellectual capacity of the patient remains essentially intact. Associationists regard intellectual activity as a function of large areas of the brain working as a whole. Most importantly, associationists regard intelligence as located outside the region bound by the language centers (Benton, 1981).

The *cognitive* school rejects the idea that thought and language are separate entities. According to Benton, Armand Trousseau first challenged the idea that thought could be largely unimpaired in aphasia. Trousseau believed that intelligence always was "lamed" in aphasia patients (Trousseau, 1865). He challenged the belief that language simply expresses thought in adults. The cognitive school took a more holistic approach to neuropathologies of speech and language.

John Hughlings Jackson was the first author to systematically study the patient's "psyche." In this dimension of the study of aphasia and related disorders, Jackson was a pioneer. For the first time, patients suffering from neurogenic communication disorders were viewed in a comprehensive manner that did not include the artificial separation of thought, speech, language, and the patient's psyche. He proposed a unitary, psychological approach to brain functioning (Benson, & Ardila, 1996). Jackson fused thought, language, and the individual's intent in communicating to the study of aphasia and related disorders.

Jackson also applied the concept of *inner speech* to the study of neurogenic communication disorders. He believed that all forms of speech were similar and that inner speech—internal monologues—occur with the same structure as other propositional utterances. Jackson believed it was artificial to consider the utterances spoken to someone else as basically different from the utterances spoken to ourselves (Sies, 1974).

Weisenburg and McBride (1935) were concerned with more than speech responses and neurology. They noted that aphasia affects the patient's reactions to practical and social situations. Although they did not identify complex personality changes in their patients, they did view aphasia as a syndrome inclusive of attitudinal and emotional changes.

Holistic theories of neuropathologies of speech and language were furthered by Kurt Goldstein. Goldstein is best known for postulating an *abstract-concrete imbalance* in aphasic patients' performance of reasoning tasks. Goldstein theorized that the aphasic patient has specific deficiencies in maintaining an *abstract attitude*. This loss of abstract attitude was present not only in language but in nonverbal performance tasks, such as sorting colors and classifying objects (Goldstein, 1924, 1948, 1952, 1959).

Goldstein was influenced by Gestalt psychology and consequently viewed aphasia and related disorders from a broad theoretical perspective. Goldstein's Gestalt psychology background provided a basis for his initial theories into the aphasic patient's ego. Goldstein viewed the aphasic patient as one suffering from a concrete attitude, bound to immediate experience, and lacking initiative and spontaneity (Schuell, Jenkins, & Jimenez-Pabon, 1964).

Joseph Wepman (1962) discussed the effects of neurogenic communication disorders on the patient's ego and self-concept, stating that "In every instance of brain damage there appears to be some degree of ego weakness and disruption of the self-concept" (p. 207). A patient with a weak or negative self-concept is likely to have narrowed or distorted perceptions and seek to defend himself or herself (Stuart, 2001a). According to Wepman, the patient must reorganize his or her self-concept and realistically assess his or her strengths and weaknesses. He writes, "The self-concept evolved must be in terms of the patient as he is, facing the reality of his condition and leaving the 'ghost of the past' that so often haunts him" (Wepman, 1962, p. 207). Wepman considered aphasia not only a language disorder but a psychological impairment as well. Indeed, the disturbance affects the patient's entire personality (Brumfitt, 1996).

Wepman (1962) and Wepman and Jones (1961, 1966) considered aphasia to be a *regression* in linguistic and cognitive functioning. According to the *linguistic regression theory*, the speechlessness of an infant reportedly corresponds to the most severe category of language disturbance: global aphasia. The stage of language development in which the child acquires vocabulary correlates with semantic aphasia. Syntactic aphasia roughly correlates with the grammatical acquisition stages of the child. They believed that the stages of recovery from aphasia should parallel these stages of language development.

A.R. Luria (1958, 1964, 1966, 1970, 1974) took exception with the linguistic regression theory and extended the argument to psychological reactions. He suggested that pathological states of the brain do not return the individual to stages of development he or she has previously passed; the effects of learning and experience are too strong. The patient's previous experiences cannot leave him or her unchanged, even after extensive brain damage. According to Luria, voluntary activity does not originate from "primordial" properties; the human experience is a process of transformation that leaves the adult unique and psychologically different from the child.

Russell Brain and Macdonald Critchley are considered pioneers in studying the neurology of aphasia and related disorders. However, they also appreciated the importance of the psychology of the patient (Sies, 1974). Brain (1965) concluded that aphasia is more than a neurological event; it also must be considered on a psychological level. Critchley (1970) explored the use of inner symbols by the aphasic patient and postulated the existence of a grammar to internal monologues.

Geschwind (1967) studied naming errors in aphasic patients and has been in the forefront of localizing language disturbances. Geschwind identified several types of aphasia, including *hysterical anomia* (difficulty remembering words, especially nouns) occurring as a manifestation of hysteria or malingering. Hysterical anomia may be the only abnormality presented by the patient, or it may occur as one symptom of a more complicated hysterical syndrome. In malingering, the patient's goal in faking illness is driven by external incentives (Frank, 1998).

J. Sarno (1981) discussed the need for a logical way to address the psychology of neurogenic communication disorders and suggested ground rules for a "science of emotions" for neurogenic communication disorders. Categorical separation of groups for study should include "patients with unilateral stroke (with the lesion in the distribution of one vessel only), space-occupying tumors, invasive tumors, missile wounds, head trauma with focal lesions (lacerations, loss of substance, intracerebral hemorrhage, peridural hemorrhage), head trauma without focal lesions and with coma" (Sarno, J., 1981, p. 481). Although etiology certainly can affect the psychology of these disorders, separating them into these small subgroups too narrowly restricts them for theoretical utility. This method offers too many categories to use successfully in the model of psychological adjustment provided in this book.

Jon Eisenson has been in the forefront of appreciating the psychological effects of aphasia. He states, "We would consider it surprising if an individual who has incurred a cerebral insult and associated aphasic disturbances did not undergo consequent changes in personality" (Eisenson, 1984, p. 87). According to Eisenson, an impairment of language affects the manner in which the personality manifests and, there are disruptions in the capacity for planning. Those who make good recoveries are those who adjust to the brain damage, and those who do not reach their potential are hindered by their premorbid inclinations and ego involvement. Eisenson explained the role of ego involvement in the aphasic patient who does not make appreciable improvement with ordinary motivation: "Their inclination, their needs, their interpretations, rather than those of their cultural environment, become the dominant ones. Thus, verbal expressions have limited meanings and restricted significance" (p. 91).

Aphasia may be more accurately defined as a "disorder of a person" than a "disorder of language" (Sarno, M., 1991). A holistic approach is warranted for those patients with personality and emotional dysfunctions associated with neurogenic communication disorders. The diagnosis and treatment of aphasia and related disorders are dynamic processes. The fact that these disorders evolve in type and severity over time requires ongoing re-evaluation not only of the speech and language symptoms, but also of their important psychological aspects.

Leonard LaPointe (1997) has proposed that aphasia and related disorders should be understood in the context of adapting to chronic illness. Adaptation and accommodation to chronic illness involves going from uncertainty to regaining wellness through taking charge, setting goals, seeking closure, and attaining mastery over the illness. Of special importance in adapting to these serious illnesses is the support and encouragement provided by family and friends (Scott & Tanner, 1990; Baker & Tanner, 1990). The importance of all members of the rehabilitation team working together on psychiatric considerations is emphasized by Frank (1998).

Contemporary neuroscientists use new techniques for studying the brain that have increased the rate of learning about its functions (Ryalls & Behrens, 2000). These include computed tomography (CT), magnetic resonance imaging (MRI), single photon tomography (SPECT), positron emission tomography (PET), and functional magnetic resonance imaging (fMRI). Research conducted with these new technologies has significant implications for theoretical models into the diagnosis, treatment, and prognosis of all aspects of neurogenic communication disorders (George, Vikingstad, & Cao, 1998). As a result, the localization movement is not dead, but it has changed and the battles rage on. There have been refinements in the armament of the academic war, but many issues remain stubbornly present. The nature of aphasia and related disorders is resistant to consensus. To know these neuropathologies of speech and language is to understand the essence of human thought.

Heilman and Valenstein (1993) have noted that there are many valid approaches to the study of the brain and no morally and intellectually sound ones should be neglected. Many issues that historically have prompted heated debates among teachers, researchers, and clinicians continue to be argued. In fact, Benson (1993) observed that the discipline of aphasiology was born from the long simmering debate over localized versus holistic explanations of functions in the brain. Rarely has the study of these disorders been free from controversy, and the psychology of them is no exception.

Multiple Determinants

Current models of personality theory and emotional disorders involve *multiple determinants*. Psychiatry attempts to explain personality disorders, behavioral problems, and emotional reactions from psychoanalytic, social-interpersonal, and psycho-organic models. The thrust of current psychiatric research involves the psycho-organic models, but many practicing psychiatrists are eclectic in their approaches to treatment (Gerstenberger, personal communications, 1987). Ongoing evaluation involves the application of appropriate treatments that frequently include a combination of approaches. Psychopharmacological agents are used with psychotherapies and improvement of social relationships to treat a variety of psychological dysfunctions (Gerstenberger, personal communications, 1990).

Based on the historical contributions of researchers and theorists reviewed in this chapter, the emotional, behavioral, and personality changes in neurogenic communication disorders can be viewed from this multiple etiological framework. As will be discussed in subsequent chapters of this book, an eclectic approach to understanding them is appropriate.

CHAPTER

2

The Big Three Neurogenic Communication Disorders and Quality of Life

"Every new adjustment is a crisis in self-esteem."

—Eric Hoffer

Awakening

Your eyes slowly open. As the fluorescent light from the room gradually penetrates your brain, you feel a crisp sheet covering your body and see a multitude of beeping, buzzing, and dripping machines, clearly hospital in origin. The sterile white ceiling stares back at you, coldly indifferent to your plight. In an adjacent room, you hear doctors and nurses talking, conferring, ordering, and prescribing. Their words seem foreign and strange. In a blur of confusion, you fight to remember what brought you to this room. You have a vague recollection of a fall to the kitchen floor. You have other blurred images of an ambulance, a gurney, a blood pressure cuff, and flashing lights.

You feel sensors patched to your chest and arm, and a prickly needle penetrating a vein. You try to move your right arm but to no avail. Your right arm muscles appear oblivious to your commands. To help them, you enlist the services of your left arm, but movement is aborted abruptly by a tightly tied restraint. You try to roll over to ease the back pain, but that too is futile. Your right leg will not move, clearly in cahoots with your stubborn arm.

Your mouth is as dry as an Arizona dust storm, and you feel a cloud of fear engulf you. You sense danger and succumb to an all-encompassing feeling of impending doom. Sweat appears on your brow. Something terrible has happened, and you know you must escape this danger. But physical escape is not an option. The path to safety is blocked by paralysis and restraints. You try and try again to escape this danger, but finally you give up and close your eyes. A woman in a white uniform utters a string of words you are incapable of understanding. You slip into the sanctuary of sleep as the nurse's word, "agitated", echoes in your mind.

Before exploring the psychology of neurogenic communication disorders, it is necessary to define and describe them. A clear understanding and a delineation of these complex communication disorders are required prior to discussing coping methods and quality of life. What follows is a review of the major neurogenic communication disorders, their etiology and prominent symptoms. Although the reader can find more detailed coverage of them in other texts, the salient aspects considered important to understanding their psychology are provided.

The three major communication disorders resulting from injury to the brain and/or nervous system are *aphasia, apraxia of speech,* and the *dysarthrias.* They are referred to as the "big three" neurogenic communication disorders (Tanner, 1999). While these disorders can occur alone, they are often seen together. They are further divided into those that impair the fabric of language (aphasia) and those that are primarily motor speech disorders (apraxia of speech and the dysarthrias). Although several classification systems of the neuropathologies of speech and language exist, in this book they are classified in the Darley tradition (Darley, 1982; Darley, Aronson, & Brown, 1975). This system is used because it clearly separates the motor speech disorders from those that disrupt language. Such a distinction is important because of the role language plays in the utilization of some coping styles and psychological defense mechanisms. Duffy (1995) found the following percentages of neurogenic communication disorders at the Mayo Clinic in Rochester, Minnesota from 1987 to 1990: 46.3% dysarthria, 27.1% aphasia, and 4.6% apraxia of speech.* Other cognitive-linguistic and neurogenic speech disorders accounted for 13.0% and 9.0% of the cases, respectively.

Aphasia

Aphasia is a language disorder that results from brain damage. It is not a speech disorder; it is an acquired pathology of language (Darley, 1982). For the purposes of this book, *language* is defined as the *multimodality* encoding, decoding, and manipulation of symbols for the purposes of verbal thought and/or communication. Language modalities include speaking, understanding what is spoken, reading, writing, and the ability to use and understand gestures and numerical symbols (see Figure 1). The severity of aphasia can range from complete loss of language to mild word-finding problems.

*The figure for apraxia of speech may be significantly higher depending on the definition and classification of aphasic disorders used.

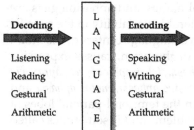

FIGURE 1 Modalities of language.

There are certain aspects of aphasia that must be considered before discussing the way people cope with it. The following are salient aspects of this language disorder:

1) Aphasia is a *multimodality* disorder. Although certain brain injuries can result in only the inability to read, to write, to speak, or to gesture, the syndrome of aphasia crosses all avenues of communication. A particular patient may have major difficulties in only one modality of communication, but he or she will also have impairments that affect other avenues (see Figure 2). Sometimes it takes detailed testing to discover these disruptions, but they are usually present.

2) Aphasia results from brain damage, usually in the left hemisphere. Most people have language located primarily in the left hemispheres of their brains. When aphasia occurs because of damage to the right hemisphere, these patients have *crossed aphasia* or *nondominant aphasia*.

3) Typically, aphasiologists divide aphasia into *expressive* and *receptive* categories. The expressive aspects of aphasia are spoken language, writing, and communicating with expressive gestures. The receptive aspects are understanding the words spoken by others, reading, and understanding the gestures of others. The ability to do simple arithmetic also involves both expression and reception of information using numerical symbols. In neurogenic communication disorders, the inability to write, read, and do simple arithmetic are called *agraphia*, *alexia*, and *acalculia*, respectively.

COMMUNICATION

Speaking..............	A	..............Listening
Listening..............	P	..............Speaking
Reading..............	H	..............Writing
Writing	A S	..............Reading
Gestures..............	I	..............Gestures
Arithmetic..............	A	..............Arithmetic

FIGURE 2 Aphasia cuts across all avenues of communication.

The expressive disorders go by several names, and aphasiologists are not consistent in their usage. There is considerable variability in the specific sites identified as the expressive and receptive language centers of the brain. Damage to *Broca's area*, in the frontal lobe of the brain, causes expressive problems and is sometimes called *Broca's aphasia, telegraphic speech, apraxia of speech, nonfluent aphasia, predominantly expressive aphasia, motor aphasia* and *anterior aphasia*. Damage to *Wernicke's area*, in the temporal-parietal lobes of the brain (Zemlin, 1998), causes receptive problems and is sometimes called *Wernicke's aphasia, jargon aphasia, fluent aphasia, predominantly receptive aphasia, sensory aphasia* and *posterior aphasia*. Severe or complete damage to both areas of the brain is called *global aphasia, irreversible aphasia syndrome* or *complete aphasia* (see Figure 3). Naming, the core deficiency in aphasia, appears to be represented throughout the brain (Ryalls & Behrens, 2000).

4) When interacting with aphasic persons, attention must be given to the input and output modalities. There are several ways of presenting information to a patient and a number of ways he or she can respond. For example, requests can be written or verbal, and the patient's responses can be gestural or verbal.

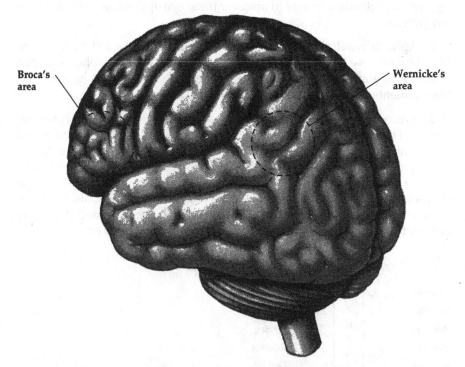

FIGURE 3   Approximate boundaries of expressive and receptive speech and language centers of the brain.

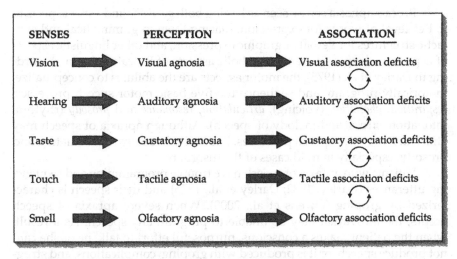

FIGURE 4 Senses and corresponding agnosias.

5) Each of the senses (vision, hearing, taste, touch, smell) have perceptual aspects that can be impaired. The perceptual disorders are referred to as the *agnosias*. In the broadest definition of the word, agnosia means lack of recognition (Benson & Ardila, 1996). Unlike aphasic disturbances, agnosias are usually modality specific and do not cross all avenues of communication. They are breakdowns in information processing occurring between the senses and associative functions of the cortex (see Figure 4). Auditory-acoustic and visual agnosias are the most important perceptual disorders to be considered in neurogenic communication disorders. Visual and auditory perception play important roles in reading and auditory comprehension. The presence of tactile agnosia is a special consideration for vision-impaired patients who use Braille.

Apraxia of Speech

Apraxia of speech is a motor speech programming disorder that often occurs in aphasia. It results from damage to Broca's area of the brain, which is in the frontal lobe of the left hemisphere of most right-handed individuals. Apraxia of speech is often an aspect of Broca's aphasia. Depending on the degree of injury to Broca's area, and the tracts leading to and from it, Broca's aphasia often has this motor speech programming component. Pure apraxia of speech is rare and results from damage to Broca's area proper (and the tracts leading to and from it), which is smaller than the area damaged in Broca's aphasia.

Broca's aphasia can be seen as having both *symbolic* and *motor* aspects to it. Retrieval of words for expression, placing them in grammatical and syntactic structures for verbal or graphic expression, and other linguistic aspects of expressive language are the symbolic aspects of Broca's aphasia. According to Darley et al. (1975), the motor aspects are the abilities to conceptualize, motorically program, and sequence the five basic motor speech processes: *respiration, phonation* (voicing), *articulation, resonance* and *prosody* (rhythm, intonation, stress, and melody of speech). Although apraxia of speech may affect all five motor speech processes, it is limited usually to articulation and prosody, especially in mild cases of the disorder.

Patients with apraxia of speech have trouble programming and sequencing utterances (Darley, 1982; Darley et al., 1975) and their speech is characterized by groping (Owens et al., 2000). When severe apraxia of speech occurs, the individual may be unable to program any speech. As a result, when the patient makes a conscious, purposeful effort to talk, he or she cannot produce speech, or it is produced with groping, complications, and struggle. However, when speech is attempted without forethought, it can sometimes be produced easily and clearly; this is called automatic speech. Profanity, for example, is sometimes uttered automatically in patients with apraxia of speech.

Apraxia of speech is usually caused by vascular disturbances such as a stroke (Duffy, 1995). It is often seen initially in brain injuries, but because of the reduction of swelling of the brain and other factors, it disappears or is reduced significantly. For many patients with neuropathologies of speech and language, it is a transitory disorder.

The Dysarthrias

The dysarthrias affect, to various degrees, the motor aspects of speech production, impacting the strength, speed, timing, direction, and range of motor speech movements (Owens et al., 2000; Darley et al., 1975) The dysarthrias are categorized based on the type and extent of the paralysis that exists (Darley et al., 1975). There are six generally recognized categories of dysarthria with common acoustic-perceptual features (see Table 1):

Flaccid dysarthria is the result of damage to lower motor neurons. Typically, with this type of dysarthria, the muscles of speech are weak and limp.

Spastic dysarthria is the result of bilateral upper motor neuron damage. In spastic dysarthria, the muscles of speech are tight and weak, and range of motion tends to be limited. In addition, Duffy (1995) has identified unilateral upper motor neuron dysarthria. It results in weakness on the opposite side of the body and the resulting speech characteristics.

TABLE 1 Dysarthria Categories

Type of Dysarthria	Neurological Deficit	Prominent Speech Pathologies
Flaccid	Lower Motor Neurons	Hypernasality Distorted and omitted phonemes Breathy voice quality
Spastic	Bilateral Upper Motor Neurons Unilateral Upper Motor Neurons	Harsh or hoarse voice quality Distorted phonemes Assimilated hypernasality
Ataxic	Cerebellum	Assimilated hypernasality Prosodic disturbances Distorted phonemes
Hypokinetic	Extrapyramidal System	Slow rate of speech Voice and articulation tremor Reduced volume
Hyperkinetic	Extrapyramidal System	Prosodic disturbances Unwanted sounds that occur quickly or slowly
Mixed	Multiple Systems	Two or more of the above pathologies occurring simultaneously, or changes in one type over time.

Ataxic dysarthria is the result of damage to the *cerebellum* and the tracts leading to and from it. The cerebellum is responsible for refining and coordinating muscular movements. Patients with ataxic dysarthria often have explosive, ill-coordinated, and jerky speech.

Hypokinetic dysarthria is seen primarily in Parkinson's disease and results from damage to the *extrapyramidal system*. Patients with hypokinetic dysarthria speak at an abnormally slow rate, often with tremors, and have weak voices.

Hyperkinetic dysarthria occurs in two forms. Quick hyperkinetic dysarthria results from damage to the *extrapyramidal system* and involves unwanted movements that happen rapidly, such as tics and jerks. When these unwanted movements affect the muscles of speech production, they create the unwanted sounds typical of this type of extrapyramidal system disorder. Slow hyperkinetic dysarthria is characterized by unwanted movements that occur slowly. It is also a result of *extrapyramidal system* dysfunction. Many patients with slow hyperkinetic dysarthria have slow, writhing movements that blend into one another, and their speech reflects this movement disorder.

Mixed dysarthria occurs when two or more of the above dysarthrias exist simultaneously. Mixed dysarthria is also present when the nature or the type of dysarthria changes over time. Approximately 50% of all dysarthrias are mixed.

Neurogenic Communication Disorders and Traumatic Brain Injury

As will be discussed in the following etiology section, neurogenic communication disorders can result from traumatic injury to the brain. The site, extent, and nature of the traumatic brain injury (TBI) determine many of the symptoms presented by the patient. There are three factors to be considered when addressing traumatic brain injuries and neurogenic communication disorders. First, a small percentage of patients primarily have their speech and language centers damaged. Because there is focalized damage, patients present with one or more neurogenic communication disorders, aphasia, apraxia of speech, and/or the dysarthrias. Their primary communication disorders resemble the aphasia, apraxia of speech, and/or dysarthrias seen in many stroke patients. These patients typically do not have arousal, orientation, behavior, judgment, and memory problems (except for word-retrieval). Second, some patients have traumatically induced brain damage, but the major speech and language centers are spared. Although these patients may have problems communicating, the fabric of language and the motor speech process remain intact. These patients primarily present with arousal, orientation, behavior, judgment, and memory problems. Third, patients can have aphasia, apraxia of speech, and the dysarthrias, compounded by arousal, orientation, behavior, judgment, and memory problems.

The common characteristic affecting communication in most patients with traumatic brain injuries is reduced or impaired consciousness. Consciousness is a person's awareness of self and his or her environment. In traumatic brain injury, impaired or reduced consciousness manifests in several ways. First, many patients have generally impaired *executive functions*, which are the abilities to set, plan, and achieve goals. Behaviorally, these impairments include problems with self-regulation, deliberation, coordination, and inhibition (Gillis, 1996). Second, patients with traumatic brain injuries are often disoriented. The disorientation can be to time, place, person, and/or situation. Third, many problems with cognition and executive functioning may be traced to memory deficits that are common in traumatic brain injuries. Both short-term and long-term memory can be impaired. Finally, traumatic brain injury often results in abnormal behaviors, including aggressiveness, sexual acting-out, and other problems with self-regulation and inhibition. The reader should consider the above when addressing the psychology of neurogenic communication disorders arising from traumatic brain injury.

The Evaluation

You are wheeled into a sterile but comfortable office. As a woman locks your wheelchair in place and engages in chitchat, you occasionally nod, provide slanted smiles, and utter "uh, huh" at the end of her statements, although only fragments of her speech are understood by you. The next hour is spent pointing to pictures, opening your mouth widely, writing, sticking out your tongue, and putting small red circles below large green squares. Scores of your responses, actions, and behaviors are noted carefully by the clinician. At the end of this emotionally draining hour, you are painfully aware of every defect, deficit, deficiency, deviation, and disorder in your once-normal ability to communicate. Despair huddles on the horizon as you begin to let the reality of your predicament set in.

In the report, the words "spastic dysarthria" label the inability to make your vocal cords vibrate easily and freely; your voice sounds as though hands are tightly choking your neck. So, too, do those medical words describe your tongue's slow, sluggish, and restricted movements. The sounds of speech, in the past so easily and automatically produced, are now made with distortions, slurs, and imprecision. Your speech muscles are weak, sluggish participants in the act of talking. Paralyzed muscles make your face rigid and, even when you can force a phoney smile, they betray your intent.

"Apraxia of speech" in the diagnostic report could better be called impotence—verbal impotence. As occasional words surface to your mind's ear, attempts to utter them are met with resistance. Try as you will, you can't seem to remember how to shape the air coming from your lungs into speech. The in and out of breathing resists formation into words. When you attempt a word, when you carefully think about its creation, you fail to complete or even start the act. It is as though the word has no trigger to fire it into existence. You feel not confused but perplexed. When flawed words emerge from your mouth, they cause your stomach to tighten. You feel out of control. It is frightening to have speech muscles with minds of their own. What is even more perplexing is the occasional utterance that flows from your mouth with ease. Like swear words that surface when your thumb is crushed by a hammer, these automatic utterances are programmed into existence when no thought is given to them. The clinician notes the presence of "automatic" speech on your report. What has not been noted is your overwhelming sense of impotence, the loss of psychological integrity and completeness of what was once you.

"Aphasia." A rose by any other name would still have thorns capable of piercing your sense of self. Where have the words gone? Where are the lost verbal trains of thought stationed? It is as though a vacuum has sucked away so many of the little and large words that once resided in your mind. What has happened to the readin', writin', and 'rithmetic you learned so many years ago in school?

As you stare intently at the nameless object carefully placed on the table by the clinician, you try and try to remember its handle. Oh sure, you know it is for grooming. With your left hand, you could easily grasp it and pull it through your hair. Its color, shape, and function are familiar, but its name escapes you. "Tooth?" No, that didn't sound right. "Brush?" No, well, maybe. "Comb." It is a "comb"! One down, thousands to go. As the hour crawls on, you confront one failure after another, while only occasionally satisfying the demanding clinician.

> Point to the fork.
> Show me the one used for eating.
> Read this word.
> Write the name of this, that, and the other thing.
> Fill in the blank.
> Complete this sentence.
> Remember this word.
> Construct this sentence.
> Choose the correct one.
> Tell me.
> Speak to me.
> Talk. Talk. Talk.

Finally, the evaluation and psychological trauma are over. Whew! Now, you will be defined, described, and diagnosed. The hows, whats, whens and wheres of rehabilitation will be fit neatly into the Medicare and HMO service standards. Fortunately for you, and unfortunately for the diagnostic report, your communication disorders and your feelings about them will change and evolve. Some of what was discovered today will be irrelevant next week, and much of the report will be obsolete next month. But let the games begin. You now have a new identity, a new role. You are now just one of many patients to the therapist. Feelings of inferiority build.

Etiology of the Big Three Neurogenic Communication Disorders

Strokes are the third leading cause of death in the United States (Owens et al., 2000). They are also the primary cause of neurogenic communication disorders. Strokes result from either *occlusive* or *hemorrhagic* interruptions of the flow of blood to the brain. Occlusive strokes occur when there is a blockage or restriction of an artery. When blood cannot get to the brain tissue, irreversible brain damage occurs. Hemorrhagic strokes occur when a blood vessel in the brain bursts, often because of high blood pressure. Not only do hemorrhages result in an interruption of the flow of blood to the designated parts of the brain, they also can cause it to be spilled into the cranial cavity. This can cause *increased cranial pressure* or ICP, sometimes called *increased intracranial pressure* (IICP). Increased cranial pressure can cause changes in the patient's speech and language behaviors, along with other medical and psychological complications. If the speech and language centers are deprived of their normal blood flow, the stroke survivor will experience one or more neurogenic communication disorders.

Neurogenic communication disorders caused by traumatic brain injuries are classified as *open* or *closed*. An open-head injury occurs when a missile, usually a bullet, enters the brain. Closed-head injuries are more common and are usually a result of motor vehicle accidents (MVAs) or falls. As reported previously, patients with traumatic brain injuries frequently suffer from behavior problems, memory deficits, and disorientation that go beyond the problems they experience with communication. These problems also interfere with communication and can create problems with making an accurate diagnosis of symptoms (Culbertson, Tanner, Peck, & Hooper, 1998).

A variety of diseases and infections of the brain can cause communication disorders. Cancerous tumors of the brain, nonmalignant growths, infections, and progressive diseases can interfere with the ability to speak or to understand the speech of others. Neurogenic communication disorders can also be caused by surgeries to remove brain tumors because efforts to gain access to them may result in damage to the speech and language centers.

Psychological Cause and Effect

Several factors related to etiology can affect the psychology of neurogenic communication disorders. The following are guidelines derived from large groups of patients, and there will be exceptions on an individual basis.

1. Traumatic brain injury tends to be associated with cognitive, memory, learning, and orientation deficits not typically seen in strokes.

2. Initially, open- and closed-head injuries tend to present with similar psychological symptoms, but as time passes, they diverge in their nature and the way they are presented.
3. Traumatic brain injuries often present with two types of brain damage that can directly cause a variety of psychological reactions. One set of symptoms is related to the site of the impact (*coup*) and the other with the recoil and impact of the brain within the skull (*contra coup*). With many patients, there is also axonal shearing and tearing.
4. Increased intracranial pressure and/or midline shifts of the brain within the cranial cavity are often associated with more spontaneous recovery and the disappearance of psychological symptoms.
5. Medications, especially those to eliminate seizures, often influence the patient's speech and language abilities and his or her psychological status. Approximately 20% of aphasic patients have some seizure activity (Owens et al., 2000).

Quality of Life Issues

For many patients, the psychological reactions to aphasia, apraxia of speech, and the dysarthrias are so prevalent and pervasive that they can be considered part of the syndrome of these disorders. Agitation, fear, anxiety, confusion, panic attacks, depression, ego restriction, withdrawal, and crying can be as much a part of these disorders as the word-finding difficulties, tip-of-the-tongue behaviors, slurred speech, reading deficits, or the understanding problems. For many patients the first step in overcoming these disorders is learning to adjust to a host of unwanted and frightening changes. Because of these factors, all clinicians who treat these patients must understand that the psychology of neurogenic communication disorders is as important as their neurology. While there is little clinicians can do to change the neurological damage, much can be done to help the patient cope and adjust to his or her limitations brought about by it. The clinician's actions can directly improve the patient's quality of life.

Several considerations go into assessing a person's quality of life. Many generalities have been made about this important aspect of living. Lawton (1991) defines quality of life in a multidimensional framework inclusive of both subjective and objective criteria (see Figure 5). According to this model, there are four critical domains: *objective environment, behavioral competence, perceived quality of life*, and *psychological well-being*. The objective environment significantly affects a person's quality of life. The environment must meet basic needs and supply the materials necessary to thrive because it serves as a foundation for self-actualization. Behaviorally, the patient must have the competence to interact with and exercise basic control over his or her environment. Perceived quality of life is the assessment the individual has about

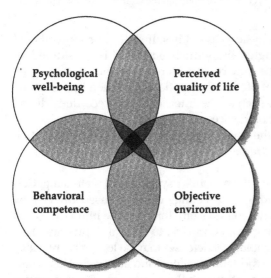

FIGURE 5   Lawton's conceptual model of quality of life. (Courtesy Slack Publishing Company)

his or her existence. It is a subjective judgment about satisfaction with life in general. Finally, quality of life is dependent on the person's psychological well-being. In Lawton's model, these four critical domains interact with each other.

For individuals with neurogenic communication disorders, the objective environment can be dramatically influenced by institutionalization. For the patient confined to a long-term rehabilitation center or nursing home, the quality of the institution has a major influence on all aspects of his or her life. From the taste and nutritional value of the food to the recreational activities supplied by the facility, the institution plays a major role in the patient's quality of life. Even for patients who are not institutionalized, the nature of the home environment, competency of the home health agency, and the availability of community services for the disabled play important roles in the quality of their lives.

Behavioral competence, particularly with regard to mobility and communication, is an important issue. Communication abilities dictate the potency and depth of social interaction. To illustrate the importance of communication on quality of life, MacNeil, Weischselbaum, & Pauker, (1981), in a study addressing laryngeal cancer and treatment options, found that the majority of subjects were willing to trade off life expectancy in order to retain the ability to speak. The patient's freedom of mobility affects his or her independence. Some patients are confined to bed while others enjoy relatively unimpeded mobility. Also, quality of life for patients with neurogenic communication disorders can be affected by their preconceived notions and stereotypes about the nature of communication disorders and physical disabilities. It should be remembered that quality of life issues are highly individualized. What is considered an impoverished existence for some may be considered rich and rewarding by others. In addition, the quality of life of many patients has been improved by modern technological advances such as the Internet, video recorders, digital hearing aids, and voice recognition devices.

There are three aspects to the psychology of neurogenic communication disorders, and each can have a dramatic effect on the patient's quality of life (see Figure 6).

First, brain injury itself affects the patient's psychological well-being. Certain thoughts, behaviors, attitudes, and feelings can be caused directly by injury to the patient's brain and nervous system. Injury to the brain can result in psychological reactions ranging from euphoria to clinical depression. Second, some coping styles and psychological defenses may no longer be available to protect a patient from negative thoughts, feelings, and attitudes. This is particularly true of patients who have completely lost language. Those defenses that are primarily verbal in nature can be impaired, leaving the patient without habitual methods of adjusting to the stresses of the disorder. Also, some patients may use immature, radical, or neurotic defenses as the stress levels increase. Third, most patients grieve over losses that have occurred. A host of unwanted changes results in predictable stages of adjustment for the patient. The influence of each factor on the psychology of neurogenic communication disorders varies among individual patients (see Figure 7).

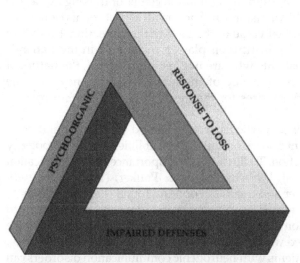

FIGURE 6   Three aspects of the psychology of neurogenic communication disorders.

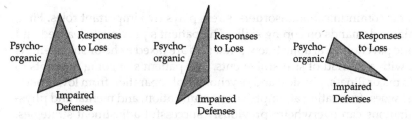

FIGURE 7   Variable influences of the three factors in the psychology of neurogenic communication disorders.

Stress and Neurogenic Communication Disorders

Stress is a core aspect of all major neurogenic communication disorders. The stressors associated with neurogenic communication disorders are varied and unique to each patient, and they can significantly affect quality of life. Listed below are common stressors associated with aphasia and related disorders.

Experiencing a medical emergency.

Suffering a serious neurological event.

Being psychologically separated from loved ones due to a communication disorder.

New relationships with doctors, nurses, and therapists.

Word-finding deficits.

Tip-of-the-tongue behaviors.

Medications.

Slurred speech.

Difficulty understanding the speech of others.

Undergoing MRI, CT, and other diagnostic tests.

Physical separation from loved ones for long periods.

Medical expenses.

Problems doing simple arithmetic.

Reading deficits.

Impairments with walking, eating, dressing, and going to the bathroom.

The knowledge that you have experienced "brain damage."

A particular person's reaction to stress is determined by the degree and chronicity of it, as well as by personality traits such as flexibility, perfectionism, compulsivity, and ambition (Duffy, 1995). When it comes to adapting to neurogenic communication disorders, stress plays two important roles. First, stress places demands on coping skills. The patient's previously learned and automatic psychological adjustment strategies are taxed as he or she attempts to cope with a myriad of stressful events. The patient's ongoing attempts to adjust to major illness, physical and psychological separation from loved ones, financial woes, frustrating attempts at communication, and mental and physical limitations can overwhelm previously successful adjustment strategies. Stress is, therefore, a risk factor in major depression (Frank, 1998). Stuart (1998) notes that the average depressed person reports three times as many important life events during the six months prior to the onset of the clinical depression than did normal subjects. Over time, the cumulative effects of the unwanted changes can exceed the patient's ability to adjust to them.

Second, the inability to cope can also be a stressor. The patient's slow, frustrating, and often unsuccessful ability to adjust can create a perception that the brain injury has eliminated his or her previously successful coping abilities. Particularly in the case of depression, this can lead to overwhelming feelings of helplessness and hopelessness. Some patients have not only been overwhelmed by stress, but they have the feeling that the brain injury itself has eliminated the possibility of ever regaining psychological stability.

When addressing the relative influence of the patient's brain injury, coping styles, psychological defenses, reaction to loss, and the role stress plays in all of them, the clinician must ask certain questions (see Figure 8).

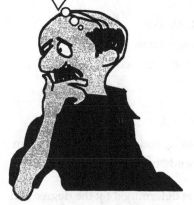

Where do I start?
What should I look for?
Why do I think this is a problem?
When should I intervene?

FIGURE 8   The what, where, why, and whens of clinical decision making.
(Courtesy Slack Publishing Company)

Where to start, what to look for, and when to intervene are basic questions every clinician must ask (Bridge & Twible, 1997). Most importantly, the clinician should assess why a patient's psychological adjustment is considered a problem and what role it plays in the four aspects of his or her quality of life. The following chapters provide detailed information to help in this important problem-solving process.

Those Were the Days

As you stare at the muted television in your hospital room, you have the sense that too much, too fast has gone wrong with your life. You sorely miss the big and little comforts of your previous existence. You wonder if you will ever have the optimism and security you enjoyed previously. There are so many demands, so many worries. Lost is the sense of well-being you once enjoyed. When you are alone, particularly in the mornings, you wonder about your future. Will your life ever be normal again? There are so many new people, issues, schedules, buildings, procedures, and concerns. You seem awash in a stream of events you cannot control. You are tired.

3
Neurogenic Communication Disorders, Brain Injury, and Psychological Adjustment

"Language is to the mind more than light is to the eye."
—William Gibson

The localization movement summarized in Chapter 1 has provided valuable information about the psychology of neurogenic communication disorders. For decades, neuroscientists have recognized certain emotions and patterns of behaviors that frequently occur in neurogenic communication disorders. Some authors refer to them as "concomitant" aspects of aphasia, apraxia of speech, and the dysarthrias. Other authorities consider them integral features of neurogenic communication disorders. Traditionally, they have been attributed directly to the effects of brain damage. However, it should be remembered that although brain injury itself can *predispose* a patient to certain emotions and behaviors, a myriad of psychological factors may also *precipitate* and *perpetuate* them.

Catastrophic Reactions

When a patient with a neurogenic communication disorder is placed in a frustrating situation, he or she may experience extreme anxiety. Anxiety disorders include panic attacks, phobias, generalized anxiety disorder, obsessive-compulsive disorders, acute stress disorders, and post-traumatic stress syndrome (Frank, 1998). In neuropathologies of speech and language, extreme anxieties, and the thoughts and patterns of behaviors occurring with them, are called *catastrophic reactions*. The anxiety can manifest itself as irritability, crying, anger, striking-out behaviors, and withdrawal. These episodes can last from seconds to minutes (Craig & Cummings, 1995).

The frustration that prompts a catastrophic reaction, in a patient prone to it, need not be extensive. All that is necessary is that he or she believes successful performance of a task is not likely. The task may be complex, such as getting to a different room, selecting a meal, or scheduling daily activities. It may be as simple as choosing a word or, once it is chosen, saying it correctly. A bombardment of sensory stimuli can also cause a catastrophic reaction. Too much noise and clutter in a room, or other distractions, may precipitate and perpetuate catastrophic reactions in patients predisposed to them.

A catastrophic reaction has been referred to as a *psychobiological break-down* (Eisenson, 1984). This term means that not only does the patient feel bombarded by sensory stimuli and overwhelmed with impotence and the possibility of failure, he or she also has biological responses to those feelings. The responses are physiological reactions typical to anxiety and fear, such as rapid respiratory rate, increased blood pressure, hypertense muscles, sweating, and dry mouth.

Some authors have suggested that catastrophic reactions occur infrequently, but others have pointed out that not all patients display observable ones. Patients with left hemisphere brain damage, particularly in and around Broca's area, are more prone to catastrophic reactions than are those with right hemisphere damage. The fluency of speech output is also associated with catastrophic reactions. The more nonfluent the speech of the patient, the more likely he or she is to have a catastrophic reaction. Psychologically, nonfluent speech tends to be more frustrating than fluent output. The relationship of post-stroke depressive episodes and catastrophic reactions is not clear (Craig & Cummings, 1995).

Most of the biological responses in a catastrophic reaction can be viewed as an acute *flight or fight response*. Subconsciously, the patient physically prepares to flee or fight the danger. Fear and anxiety are found in the perceived threat to the basic integrity of the individual. Because the individual cannot perform as he or she once normally did, panic sets in. A panic attack occurs when the human alarm system is triggered (Laraia, 1998). The biological responses are the individual's physical preparation either to flee from the threatening situation or to physically overcome it. Catastrophic reactions result from the patient's attempts to regain control, normalcy, and psychological integrity. These patterned responses often cause even more anxiety, and the result is a cascade of negative emotions and the patient's reaction to them.

Clinically, the best method of dealing with a catastrophic reaction is to prevent it. Unfortunately, it may take one occurrence of a catastrophic reaction before it can be determined that a patient is prone to it. But once it has been determined that a patient is predisposed to a catastrophic reaction, care should be taken to limit the amount of noise, distraction, and demands placed on him or her. Once a patient has begun to have a catastrophic reaction, immediate reduction of stimuli is required, as is an avenue of escape. Escape and relief for the patient can be leaving the room, having others leave, or even allowing the bed covers to be pulled over his or her head. Additionally, certain medications can be helpful in preventing catastrophic reactions.

Many antianxiety drugs can be addictive, however, and long-term use of them is usually contraindicated.

The Feeling of Impending Doom

You like having visitors. It is usually comforting to have your children and grandchildren visit you. Today, your tiny room seems full of grandchildren teasing, touching, and terrorizing each other. Your son keeps asking if you understand him, while your daughter adjusts the sheets on your bed. Overhead, you hear the hospital public address system repeatedly call a doctor to the emergency room, and outside an industrial vacuum is howling. You hear the clink and clank of the lunch tray as it is brought to your bed, and you are lifted into a vertical eating position. The children talk louder and begin playing a game of tag in your miniature room, which appears to be getting smaller by the minute. Your son is holding a picture of a relative close to your face and demanding that you say her name. When you don't respond, he shouts the question louder and louder. Your heart is pounding. Your daughter is now putting a paper napkin to your neck, and soon spoonful after spoonful of brown puree mix will be brought to your mouth. The children, the vacuum, the noise! Why can't you remember the name of the relative? She is so familiar. Then, it all becomes too much. An alarm goes off in your mind and you begin to sweat. You repeatedly try to turn away from the relative's picture. The vacuum is roaring in your head. You must escape, but there is no route to safety. You try to push the food tray away gently, but too much force causes it to fall to the floor. More noise, and the startled looks on their faces cause you to panic. What have you done? You try to cover your head with the sheet, but your hand will not obey your wishes. Finally, a nurse enters the room and suggests to your family that you need to rest. You try to explain to them about the noise, the demands, the panic, but words fail you. You finally close your eyes and pretend to sleep.

Emotional Lability

Sometimes called *pseudobulbar emotional lability*, uncontrolled crying often occurs in patients who have had bilateral damage to the motor strips (and associated corticobulbar tracts) of the brain. Thus, some patients with spastic dysarthria cry for no apparent reason or cry too much over little things. In fact, emotional lability is not seen only when a patient cries; other emotional responses may be present, too. Some patients also laugh over minor things or at apparently inappropriate times. However, because there is more to be sad about, crying is usually the behavior seen in emotionally labile patients. These emotional behaviors can convey an impression of dementia, but they may occur without any evidence of it (Duffy, 1995).

Some authorities on the subject of emotional lability believe that crying is the physical behavior lacking emotion. To some specialists, the crying is disconnected from any true emotion or feeling. In the past, many of these specialists considered emotional lability to be an "inappropriate" emotional response, one that is out of context. Unfortunately, some people view all emotional responses by labile patients as manifestations of the brain injury, and not as the results of environmental factors or changes in the patient because of limitations caused by the disabilities. Emotional lability has also been considered as manifestation of a catastrophic reaction in patients prone to crying (Gainotti, 1989). When emotional lability occurs during speech, it can have a significant negative effect on intelligibility (Duffy, 1995).

In most patients with emotional lability, however, the crying is neither inappropriate nor lacking feeling. Labile patients have *exaggerated* emotional responses rather than *inappropriate* ones. They cry too easily and too long usually over clearly identifiable stimuli. There are three precipitators of labile crying: words, situations, and thoughts.

Highly charged and emotional words uttered by either the patient or others can set off a bout of crying. Words like "nursing home," "grandchildren," and "home" can result in crying. Visits by relatives and friends can also trigger crying. Negative thoughts, particularly about the patient's predicament, can cause emotionally labile crying behaviors. When all three of the precipitators occur together, such as a relative commenting on the likelihood of the patient ever returning home, the bout of crying can be extensive. Once the crying has begun, many patients have difficulty stopping it.

The clinical management of episodes of emotional lability includes preventing their occurrences and, if that fails, reducing the duration of them. Clinicians should be alert to the patient's emotional triggers, and when topics of discussions appear to be precipitating emotional lability, they should be shifted to more pleasant and emotionally positive subjects. Distracting the patient from negativity can help reduce a bout of emotional lability once it has begun. If behavioral management methods are unsuccessful in decreasing emotional lability, a physician's prescription for an antidepressant, or other medication, may be useful.

Crying Time, Again

"Day passes." This is the term given for your release from the confines of the nursing home, an opportunity to visit the familiar. You look forward to the opportunity to see your children and grandchildren, even if it is just for a day. Last weekend, you enjoyed the company of your daughter, and this weekend, you get to visit your son. On the drive to his house, you take in the images of the fall trees, colorful leaves falling to the ground, and the usual traffic congestion. You see his house in the distance, and as you pull into the driveway, the twins, your only grandchildren, come running to greet you. When they shout your name, you feel tears flood to your eyes. The welling of tears sets off a bout of uncontrollable crying, downright sobbing. The crying causes the twins to have startled looks on their cherubic faces, and this too feeds your crying. Try as you may, you cannot stop sobbing. The embarrassment you feel is incredible. Oh sure, you feel strong emotions about the twins, but the crying is way out of proportion. And the more you cry, it seems, the more you must cry. Finally, the crying subsides as you concentrate on the complicated requirements of moving from the passenger seat of the car to the confines of your wheelchair.

Perseveration

Perseveration is the tendency to continue an activity for a longer duration than is appropriate or warranted by the significance of the stimuli. It is like the patient gets "stuck" in a mental set or behavior pattern and cannot shift to another one. In patients with neurogenic communication disorders, the two most common types of observable perseveration are *verbal* and *graphic*.

Patients with verbal (recurrent) perseveration often repeat the same sound, word, or phrase over and over. This pattern of behavior is readily apparent during sentence completion drills. For example, when the clinician asks a patient to complete the sentence, "Knife, fork and _____," the patient will initially provide the correct word "spoon." In the subsequent sentence completion activities, the patient might also reply "spoon" to the sentences, "Red, white and _____," "The United States of _____," and "You write with a _____."

Another manifestation of verbal perseveration is *echolalia* (Eisenson, 1984), the tendency of the patient to repeat the last sound, word, or phrase spoken by someone else. It is the unsolicited repetition or partial repetition of another person's utterances (LaPointe & Katz, 1998). For example, a family member might say to a patient, "How are you today?", and the patient will automatically respond with the word, "Today." When the family member asks the patient if he or she would like to go outside, the patient would automatically respond, "Outside." The patient's train of thought is contaminated by the last word spoken. According to Benson and Ardila (1996), echolalia is a feature of many degenerative brain diseases.

Graphic perseveration is seen when the patient's writing consists of letters repeated over and over. Often these attempts at writing trail off to unintelligible, small scribbles that do not resemble the first letter. It is as though the patient cannot shift his or her hand movements from one pattern to another.

The tendency to perseverate has not been identified with a specific damaged area of the brain (Swindell, Holland, & Reinmuth, 1998). As a rule, however, the greater the brain damage, the more likely the patient is to perseverate. An organic explanation for perseveration is a lack of neurotransmitters, particularly those that inhibit neuronal activity. The lack of these chemicals is a direct or indirect result of the brain injury.

One way of understanding perseveration is to liken it to a song or melody that normal individuals sometimes cannot eliminate from their thoughts. Of course, the major differences are the increased frequency and intensity of the thoughts and behaviors in the perservatory individual. Although perseveration involves different behaviors and consequences, it can be compared to *obsessive-compulsive* disorders. The patient with perseveration is obsessed with a thought or movement pattern and compulsively engages in it. The psychological explanation for repeatedly engaging in certain behaviors is that any activity, even one clearly unsuccessful and incorrect, maintains the patient's sense of self. Some patients with obsessive-compulsive disorders engage in mental rituals (Carlat, 1999) that give them a sense of potency and are ultimately reinforcing.

Perseveration plays an important role in certain emotional disorders in some patients with aphasia, apraxia of speech, and the dysarthrias. The tendency of the patient to repeatedly engage in negative thought patterns perpetuates feelings of anxiety, depression, hopelessness, helplessness, and despair. Perseveration certainly interferes with the treatment of the psychological aspects of communication disorders because it creates a rigid mental set. Patients' flexibility of thought is necessary for them to benefit from many counseling approaches.

The very presence of perseveration interferes with the treatment of neurogenic communication disorders and has a negative influence on prognosis. Perseveration negatively interacts with aphasia and complicates therapy (Holland & Beeson, 1995). Learning, relearning, and adapting to these disorders requires flexibility of thought and action. The patient's inability to shift from one idea or behavior to another can dramatically impede rehabilitation.

Two psychological factors must be addressed, therefore, in the treatment of perseveration. First, the patient's exposure to clinical stimulation must start off slowly and increase gradually. The patient should initially be seen in a quiet room with little ambient noise and clutter, and the therapy activities should be easy and simple. Gradually, the stimuli can be increased in number and complexity. Second, the patient's successful attempts at shifting from one task to another must be rewarded immediately. The rewards should be for actual shifts in behaviors and for his or her motivation and courage to face new obstacles. The patient should be cognizant that "flexibility of thought and action" is the desired behavior and that support and encouragement will be readily provided by the clinician.

Anything is Better than Nothing

You look forward to the therapy sessions with the speech-language pathologist. You receive guidance and direction in overcoming your communication disorder, which you desperately need. The frequent verbal praise and friendly pats on the back give your sagging emotions a boost. Today, you work at writing your name, an activity performed thousands of times in the past with ease and agility. You grasp a pencil in your left hand and begin the first letter. With a sense of hope building in your mind, you see that the first letter actually resembles an English one. So, too, does the second letter of your name. But, for some reason, you cannot remember the shape of the third letter. Rather than stop, admit your failure to perform such an easy, personal task, you keep writing. The second letter appears over and over. But at least you are writing . . . doing something. Perhaps the clinician will think you just have poor penmanship, what with having to write with the left hand rather than your usual right one. The letters finally trail off into a straight line, and yet another test of your well-with-all is over. You stare at the strange scribbles. At least there is something covering the blank page.

Other Organically Based Psychological Reactions

It is difficult, if not impossible, to separate the psychological reactions seen in neurogenic communication disorders into those that clearly occur because of brain injury and those that are nonorganic in origin. In aware patients, there is always a psychological component to a significant injury to the brain and nervous system. However, certain psychological reactions have been linked to specific areas and types of brain damage. This has lead some scientists to recognize that focalized brain damage predisposes, precipitates, or perpetuates psychological reactions in certain patients. *Euphoria*, *organic depression*, *behavioral changes*, *denial of disability*, and *visual neglect* are some of the psychological conditions often attributed to specific brain injuries.

Euphoria

Some patients with neurogenic communication disorders have a heightened sense of well-being. They show indifference or even a happy-go-lucky attitude about their condition. Very little frustration with the communication disorders and co-occurring physical disabilities is evident in them. It is as though these patients do not fully appreciate what has happened to them. In addition, some patients seem to bask in the attention they receive from clinicians and others. Euphoria can be a chronic personality condition, particularly with fluent aphasic syndromes (Craig & Cummings, 1995).

Euphoria can result from functional and organic factors. It is well known that anoxia can cause euphoria. When the brain does not receive the needed oxygen, the psychological result is a heightened sense of well-being. Strokes and brain trauma result in depravation of oxygen to brain cells and can cause this sense of euphoria. However, nonorganic factors can cause or contribute to euphoria as well.

Denial of disability and other psychological defenses can result in euphoria. When a patient does not allow himself or herself to become conscious of the negative things that have happened, then only positive thoughts and feelings remain. Denial and resulting euphoria were reported by one patient who said, "I heeded only the most obvious optimistic things that were said to me and for the rest I did not hear them or came to the conclusion that they were wrong. If I had allowed myself to be given a glimpse of the truth, I believe I would have gone out of my mind" (Ritchie, 1961, pp. 35–36). Exclusion of the negative and persistent adherence to only the positive can result in a feeling of well-being. Similar euphoric patterns occur in certain religious ceremonies where the participants become so involved with uplifting thoughts and rituals that they experience a sense of euphoria. Interestingly, during this euphoric state, some church members talk in "tongues," an occurrence that has similarities to the speech seen in fluent aphasic syndromes.

Very little has been written about treating the euphoric patient with neurogenic communication disorders. Perhaps this is because the euphoric patient appears content and accepting and does not appear to be in psychological distress. Some patients with traumatic brain injuries, partially because of euphoria, must be convinced of their deficits. Unfortunately, the euphoric patient may lack motivation to engage rehabilitation. Additionally, the level of therapy participation seen in these patients may be too superficial for meaningful gains.

It should be noted that whether the euphoria is caused by organic or functional factors, the patient is not properly adjusting to his or her disabilities. The patient displaying euphoria is separated from the emotional reality of the situation. As such, gradual and supportive confrontation of the psychological ramifications of the communication disorder is a necessary prerequisite to rehabilitation. Until the patient can appreciate his or her predicament, both cognitively and emotionally, meaningful gains are not likely to occur.

Organic Depression

Patients with neurogenic communication disorders are prone to depression caused by a chemical imbalance in the brain. There are important neurophysiological changes associated with organic depression (Craig & Cummings,

1995). The chemicals that create feelings of well-being can be deficient, resulting in clinical depression. The chemical imbalance can be caused directly by the injury to specific brain cells, or it may be indirectly related to the general altered chemistry caused by the stroke, traumatic brain injury, disease, and medications used to treat them. The primary cause of depression in these patients is the chemical imbalance, and the grieving and stresses associated with the neurogenic communication disorders are secondary. In many cases, this depression is associated with anxiety. As a result of depression-anxiety, the patient may become anxious and preoccupied with body and mental changes. In most patients, the *joie de vivre* is lost. For some depressed patients, the possibility of suicide must be recognized and appropriate prevention measures taken (Benson & Ardila, 1996).

There are several successful treatments for depression. Unfortunately, for patients with significant neurogenic communication disorders, counseling and psychotherapy are not realistic treatment options. Because of their inability to express themselves, many patients with aphasia cannot benefit from the "talking" cure. Even patients with motor speech disorders are unlikely to benefit from counseling and psychotherapy because, although they can understand the speech of others, their communication deficits often prohibit them from freely expressing themselves and providing ongoing psychological feedback. However, for patients who can adequately express themselves, group speech and language therapy can be beneficial to psychological adjustment. Even nonverbal and globally aphasic patients may be able to benefit from being silent members of group therapy sessions.

Antidepressants are the best treatment for patients with prolonged organically induced depression. The patient's physician can prescribe one of the many antidepressant medications currently available. These medications have few side effects and a high success rate in reducing the duration and extent of depression. For some patients, antidepressant medication will be required permanently to adjust for the chemical imbalances. For other depressed patients with neurogenic communication disorders, antidepressants are only necessary until the brain readjusts its biochemistry.

Behavioral Changes

The behavioral changes seen in some patients with neurogenic communication disorders can range from mild personality quirks that are noticeable only to close family members and friends, to bizarre and inappropriate actions that can cause harm to the patient or others. The bizarre and inappropriate behavioral problems, often with a sexual theme, are seen more often in patients who have suffered traumatic brain injury than in those who have had a stroke.

The barely noticeable behavioral changes observed by family and friends are usually the result of a *flat affect*, in which the range of the patient's overall emotional responsiveness is narrowed. Family members observe that the patient simply does not have the responsiveness and emotions typical of him or her before the neurological damage. Sometimes, this flat affect can be a symptom of undiagnosed depression.

Many of the bizarre behavioral problems seen in these patients are the direct results of disorientation and memory deficits, things common to traumatic brain injury (Tanner, Baker, Culbertson, & Palcich, 1993; Tanner, 1987). These patterns of behavior depend on many factors, including hemispheric site of lesion. Psychologically, they occur because of the loss of regulatory functions of the personality. In traditional Freudian terms, the patient's brain injury has disrupted the superego's ability to regulate the personality. Powerful needs drive the patient, and he or she is free to act on them because of the memory deficits and disorientation. The patient cannot remember moral and behavioral admonishments, is confused about appropriateness of societal norms, and thus acts in a socially unacceptable manner. The frequency and severity of these bizarre behaviors usually decrease as the patient gains orientation and as his or her memory improves.

The treatment of behavioral problems in patients with neurogenic communication disorders requires participation of the entire rehabilitation team. Participation in direct therapy by the patient's family is also important (Währborg, 1996). Specific behavior problems need to be identified by the rehabilitation team and family and targeted for management. Consistency is important. The patient should know the specific behaviors that are appropriate and those which are inappropriate. Behavior modification programs can range from simply rewarding appropriate behaviors to discouraging those that are inappropriate. Rewarding *incompatible alternatives* to undesired behaviors is one of the best methods. Having the patient find a behavior that is incompatible with the undesired one, and rewarding it, is a positive method of treatment. In addition, some patients benefit from medications to reduce agitation and acting-out behaviors.

Anosognosia

Denial is a component of many defense mechanisms. Denial of disability is called *anosognosia*. There are many forms of anosognosia, and they are often related to damage to the parietal lobes. Right-sided parietal lobe damage tends to result in more severe and persistent anosognosia. Psychologically, the patient with anosognosia does not permit the conscious perception of disability. Also, a patient with anosognosia may fail to see his or her disability in the proper perspective (Benson & Ardila, 1996). He or she blocks the reality of the situation from consciousness.

Denial of disability may also occur in the grieving process. Denial is often the first stage in complex process of accepting unwanted change (see Chapter 5). Some authorities consider all denial a direct result of brain damage and blockage of neurotransmissions from the senses to the cortex. Extreme denial or distortion of external reality can signal psychotic thought processes (Carlat, 1999).

Denial of disability can be partial or complete. In *partial denial*, the patient is aware of selected aspects of the disability but blocks others from conscious awareness. In *complete denial*, the patient may not acknowledge that any negative medical event has occurred. For example, even though the patients may have aphasia, apraxia of speech and dysarthria, and be confined to a hospital bed because of paralysis, they will maintain that they are in the hospital for a routine medical checkup or to visit other patients.

There is often a religious or spiritual theme to denial. Religion and spirituality can have a positive or negative effect on a patient's mental health (Oakley, 1998; Huttlinger & Tanner, 1994; Tanner & Huttlinger, 1989). Patients with an *external frame of reference*, those who believe many life experiences are caused or influenced by external forces, are often passive in their denial. They deny partially or completely their disability and attribute any dysfunction to external forces. They often discount the need to participate in medical treatment because they believe God or another force will make them whole again. They deny the reality of the situation and the realities associated with recovery.

Patients with an *internal frame of reference*, those who accept personal responsibility for much of life's experiences, may overestimate the extent to which their actions can return them to normal functioning. These patients believe that through sheer will and persistence, they can completely overcome the negative things that have happened to them. They deny the extent and severity of the disability and their abilities to overcome it.

Patients who use denial extensively and persistently are unrealistic. As a result of their unrealistic perceptions about their disability, they can pose special problems in rehabilitation. First, because of denial, they may never fully confront their disability. Because they deny it exists, they are incapable of focusing attention on treatment. Second, some clinicians have a tendency to treat denial with brutal confrontation about the disability. This type of confrontation with the disability tends to deepen denial because the patient is not provided with the necessary support and encouragement to turn to less radical defenses. Third, patients who are fixed in denial threaten the rehabilitation team. Because patients in denial see no need for help from the rehabilitation specialists, these patients often create a negative relationship concerning traditional medical roles. Denying patients do not validate the role of the health care provider or the role of the patient as a willing recipient of his or her services.

What Arm?

You sit in the wheelchair looking at yourself in the full-length mirror. The hospital gown barely covers your body. You see your hair, piercing eyes, and wry smile. Your feet and legs are reflected in their true form. But you don't see the reflection of your defective arm. You manage to examine every part of your body but your useless right arm. It has been weeks since it was able to move up and down, grasp and release, pick up and drop things from your daily life. It is now slung to your body, dead weight. A remnant of function that once was. It is easier to deny its existence than to deal with its reality. You don't see it, think of it, or even acknowledge its existence. In the back of your mind, you know that you will eventually give the time and attention necessary to accept it, but not now. It is too soon. For psychological and practical purposes, it doesn't exist.

The Meaning of Jargon Aphasia

The role denial plays in jargon aphasia was postulated by Weinstein and others in their classic articles published in the 1960s and 1970s. Persistent jargon speech, which is often an aspect of receptive aphasia, is a result, at least in part, of denial of disability (Weinstein et al., 1966; Weinstein & Puig-Antich, 1974). Jargon speech seen in these patients is a result of damage to Wernicke's and adjacent areas of the left temporal-parietal lobes. Jargon results from breakdown of the phonological, grammatical, and/or semantic aspects of language. Jargon aphasia patients produce output that is fluent but meaningless. They rarely pause for acknowledgment or turn-taking in conversations (Owens et al., 2000). Some Wernicke's aphasia patients are completely unaware of their deficits due to brain damage.

However, many jargon aphasic patients persist in their meaningless output. Even when it is apparent to them that little, if any, meaningful communication has taken place, these patients continue to speak jargon. Some patients also engage in projection (see Chapter 4). They attribute the lack of meaningful communication to the listener's inability or unwillingness to understand their "perfectly normal" speech. Even when it is repeatedly apparent that their jargon output does not result in functional communication, such as obtaining a requested object or having other needs met, they persist in uttering nonsense. Some deny the fact that their output is meaningless. Many jargon aphasic patients persist in this meaningless output even though it is apparent by the actions of others that communication has not taken place. There are many factors that can account for persistent jargon speech, including the inability to monitor output, disruption to semantic processing, confusion, and memory limitations. Persistent jargon is also at least partially attributable to anosognosia, the denial of disability in many patients.

When treating jargon aphasia, it is important to gradually and gently confront the patient with the realities of his or her communication disorder. Each attempt by the patient to acknowledge the reality of the situation should be met with rewards, support, and encouragement. A patient must be aware of his or her disability to overcome it.

Case Study: "That's Not Me"

A 58-year-old, right-handed male suffered brain injury to the left temporal-parietal lobes. He presented with jargon aphasia. After several weeks in a rehabilitation center, his jargon persisted. All clinical attempts to reduce the jargon speech were unsuccessful. Every time the patient was confronted with a naming task, he would refuse to participate, at any level, in the therapy. He persistently denied his communication disorder. Time spent in speech and language therapy was unproductive.

Based on a recommendation from a psychiatrist, the patient was videotaped during therapy. Close-ups were made of him denying his word-finding deficits and use of jargon. The final video was a ten-minute demonstration of the patient's word-finding deficits and jargon output.

The patient was brought to a conference room to watch the final edited video. His wife and adult son were also present to provide support and encouragement. During the video replay, the patient was agitated and angry. At the conclusion of the showing, the clinician asked the patient what he thought of the video. Through convoluted, jargon speech, the patient clearly communicated to family and staff that he was not the person in the video, and even if it were him, there was no problem whatsoever with his communication.

The patient continued to deny his jargon speech and ultimately was discharged to home. Over time his speech improved, but he never fully accepted that he had a communication disorder.

Visual Neglect

Certain types of brain damage cause blindness in either the right or left fields of both eyes. A type of cortical or perceptual blindness, this condition is called *homonymous hemianopsia*. Clearly organic in etiology, this type of blindness is directly caused by damage to the occipital lobes or the pathways leading to and from them. For the patient, homonymous hemianopsia results in blindness in either the right or left fields of his or her visual world. However, many patients with homonymous hemianopsia also engage in *visual neglect*, which is often associated with parietal-lobe damage. Patients with this blindness will not cross the visual midline and attend to people or things in the affected side. When eating, these patients will consume the foods in only the non-affected sides of their visual fields. Women, when applying makeup, place it on only the non-affected sides of their faces. Patients engage in these behaviors even though they could turn their heads and compensate for the visual field cuts. They resist, often with fervor, any attempt to get them to acknowledge the affected side. Visual field disturbance also interferes with the ability to read.

Hemialexia is the inability to attend to one-half of a line on a printed page (Benson & Ardila, 1996). Homonymous hemianopsia also results in difficulty naming objects (Marquardt, 2000).

A psychological explanation for visual neglect is that although the blindness is a direct result of brain injury, failure to compensate for it is a manifestation of denial and avoidance. Patients with visual neglect avoid looking to the affected, disordered sides of their world because that is where threatening and negative things have happened. By avoiding confrontation with the defective sides of their world, they maintain psychological integrity and wholeness. Only through gradual steps can they learn to confront the threatening situation. With support and encouragement, systematic and gradual steps can be taken to treat the psychological effects of the homonymous hemianopsia.

Psychological Reactions and Brain Localization

As reported previously, research currently being conducted in the psychology of neurogenic communication disorders focuses on localization issues. The goal of these studies is to identify the site of the lesion with the psychological reactions observed in the patient. Scientists use sophisticated scanning instruments to find the site in the brain where certain psychological reactions and disorders occur.

What has this research discovered about brain injury, neurogenic communication disorders, and the patient's psychological reaction to them? First, because the brain operates as a whole, no one area alone is completely responsible for a psychological reaction. Therefore, it is difficult to attribute any particular psychological reaction to one area. For example, two patients can have the same areas of their brain damaged and experience dramatically different psychological reactions. One patient may experience depression, whereas another might feel a heightened sense of well-being or be indifferent to negative events that are happening to him or her.

Second, it is impossible to separate the effects of the brain injury from the patient's psychological adjustment strategies. Neuroscientists do not know whether a particular psychological reaction is the result of the brain injury or whether it is the effect of the disorder on the patient's quality of life. For example, depression in some individuals can be caused by a chemical imbalance, but depression can also be caused by stress and grief. If a patient has an injury to the brain and depression results, is it because of the brain damage or because the disability is stressful and grievous?

Listed below are broad generalities that can be made about brain injury and its psychological effects on certain patients with communication disorders (Gordon, Hibbard, & Morgenstein, 1996; Tanner, 1996; Herrmann, Barrels, & Wallesch, 1993; Herrmann & Wallesch, 1989; Gainotti, 1989; Robinson, Boston, Starkstein, & Price, 1988; Lipsey, Spencer, Rabins, & Robinson, 1986; Robinson, 1986; Robinson et al., 1985; Gordon, Hibbard, Egelko, & Diller, 1985; Sackeim & Weber, 1982; Sackeim, Greenberg, Weiman, Gur, Hungerbahler, & Geschwin, 1982; Robinson & Benson, 1981; Gasparini, Satz, Heilman, & Coolidge, 1978; Black, 1975; Weinstein & Puig-Antich, 1974; Gainotti, 1972; Weinstein, Lyerly, Cole, & Ozer, 1966; and others). It should be remembered that these generalities are for large groups of patients, and there will be individual exceptions.

1. Many of the psychological symptoms caused by brain injury are similar to the psychological reactions seen in classic (or functional) emotional disturbances. Many of the psychological reactions caused by brain injury are not substantially different from the kind of psychological reactions seen in emotionally disturbed people without brain injury.
2. Patients with left-hemisphere damage tend to have more depression and anxiety than do those with right-hemisphere brain damage. Patients with right-hemisphere damage tend to exhibit indifference, apathy, cheerfulness, or even euphoria.
3. Approximately 50% of people who have a communication disorder resulting from stroke will experience depression that will be long lasting.
4. When the brain injury is in the anterior part of the left hemisphere, as many as 70% of patients are likely to experience depression. When the injury is in posterior part of the left hemisphere, many patients have indifference, lack of awareness of disabilities, and/or euphoria.
5. Many patients with receptive aphasia have a lack of awareness of their communication disorder, and some patients engage in active denial of disability. Among Wernicke's patients, larger lesions are associated with less depression.
6. Smaller brain lesions, and those closer to the anterior part of the brain, appear to result in more awareness of the disability and resulting psychological reactions. The more aware a patient is of his or her disability, the more likely he or she will experience anxiety, frustration, and depression.
7. The more nonfluent the aphasia, the more likely the patient will have short-lived emotional outbursts, anxiety, and depression.
8. Emotional lability is caused by bilateral damage to the motor strips and associated corticobulbar tracts.

Figure 9 shows the human brain and general areas that, when damaged, are associated with certain psychological reactions in some patients with neurogenic communication disorders.

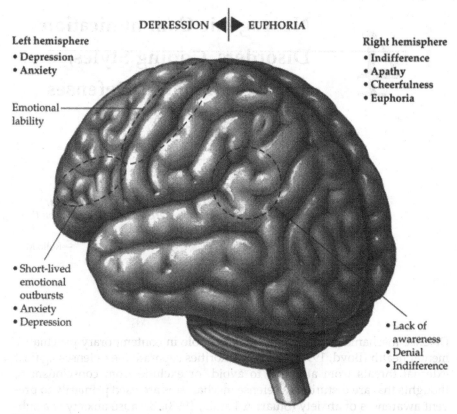

DEPRESSION ◄|► EUPHORIA

Left hemisphere
• Depression
• Anxiety

Emotional lability

• Short-lived emotional outbursts
• Anxiety
• Depression

Right hemisphere
• Indifference
• Apathy
• Cheerfulness
• Euphoria

• Lack of awareness
• Denial
• Indifference

FIGURE 9 Approximate sites in the brain associated with psychological reactions in some patients with neurogenic communication disorders.

CHAPTER

4

Neurogenic Communication Disorders, Coping Styles, and Psychological Defenses

"Anxiety is essential to the human condition. The confrontation with anxiety can relieve us from boredom, sharpen the sensitivity and assure the presence of tension that is necessary to preserve human existence."

—Rollo May

Defense mechanisms play an explanatory role in contemporary psychiatric mental health (Boyd, 1998a). Some authorities separate the defenses against external threats from attempts to avoid, or exclude from consciousness, thoughts that are disturbing. Defense mechanisms are used primarily to prevent awareness of anxiety (Stuart & Laraia, 1998). Because anxiety is a subjective individual experience (Oakley, 1998), there is little agreement about the nature of these defenses and much overlap.

There is no universally accepted list of defense mechanisms, and the mechanisms themselves are as varied as people's personalities. "It is said that coping styles and defense mechanisms are similar concepts" (Carlat, 1999, p. 62). Some coping styles and defenses are mature and have a positive effect on the psychological status of the person, while others are immature, maladaptive, neurotic, radical, or desperate attempts to cope with stressors. Mature defenses are those used by healthy people to cope with stressors. They arise from and lead to psychological health (Carlat, 1999). Maladaptive, immature, neurotic, and radical defenses are employed when stressors, and the person's ability to cope with them, become overwhelming. Unfortunately, defenses do not work effectively in all situations, and the individual develops more of them in response to increased threats (Crowe, 1997).

Patients with motor speech disorders, those neurogenic communication disorders that do not disrupt the fabric of language, should be able to use the coping styles and defense mechanisms that they previously employed. Apraxia of speech and the dysarthrias do not impair the fabric of language.

Therefore, all of the defenses, both verbal and nonverbal, remain available to the patient with apraxia of speech and the dysarthrias. Certainly, patients with motor speech disorders are confronted with major adjustment and coping challenges, but they are not impaired in using their preexisting defense mechanisms by the neurological deficit or brain injury.

The role language plays in using verbal defense mechanisms is paramount. Patients with aphasia, therefore, will have disruptions in their abilities to utilize verbal defense mechanisms (Tanner, 1999; Tanner, 1996). The degree of difficulty in using defense mechanisms depends on the extent to which language has been disrupted and on the type of aphasia. Patients with mild language deficits, those with minimal word-finding problems and deficits understanding the speech of others, should suffer only minor limitations in utilizing the verbal defense mechanisms. Conversely, patients with global or complete aphasia will be unable to engage verbal defense mechanisms because language itself has been eliminated from their cognitive processes (Tanner & Barnwell, 1994).

The following is a review of major coping styles and psychological defenses, and the degree to which language deprived patients may be able to utilize them. It is important for clinicians to comprehend the purpose of a client's defense mechanism (Crowe, 1997). Although the nature of coping styles and defense mechanisms is the subject of debate, they are used by people for psychological protection. Clinicians should encourage and support the patient's appropriate utilization of mature, adaptive defenses. Maladaptive, immature, neurotic, and radical defenses should be recognized as indications of the seriousness of the patient's attempts to deal with stressors. It also should be recognized that even mature, adaptive defenses and coping styles can be unproductive when used too much and/or too often.

Avoidance

Avoidance is innate in people and one of the simplest known defenses (Mahl, 1971). When a patient is confronted with an unpleasant or a threatening situation, and the thoughts and feelings associated with it, he or she can engage in behaviors to avoid it. By avoiding unpleasantness, the patient successfully protects himself or herself both physically and psychologically. Carlat (1999) notes that the avoiding patient may be preoccupied with the thought of rejection.

Actually, there are two ways a person can avoid unpleasantness. First, he or she can engage in *postponement*. In postponement, the patient delays confrontation of the perceived negative event and the thoughts and feelings associated with it. Excuses may be given for why he or she cannot engage in the threatening activity. Postponement temporarily provides the patient with both psychological and physical relief.

The second way a person can avoid unpleasantness is through *refusal*. When postponement is unsuccessful, the patient can flatly refuse to confront the threatening situation. In refusal, the patient physically does not allow himself or herself to engage in the negative activity. Refusal is a more extreme aspect of avoidance, but it protects and insulates the patient from threatening situations and negativity.

For patients with neurogenic communication disorders, there is much to avoid. Painful physical therapies, confinement to a hospital room, new routines and activities, and confrontation with speech and language disabilities are all situations that can result in avoidance. Avoidance, whether it is in the form of postponement or refusal, provides the patient with psychological and physical relief. Unimpaired language is not necessary to engage in avoidance. Avoidance, when used sparingly and appropriately, is an adaptive way of coping with negativity. It can provide the patient with needed respite from unnecessary negativity and allow for a reduction of stress.

Solace in the Solarium

It is pleasant to be able to get around by yourself. You have learned to move from one place to another in the wheelchair. You must pull and push with your left foot, and roll the wheel with your left hand, but you can get around. Freedom for independent movement is one of the few pleasures in your life. But the pleasant thoughts of freedom for movement are rapidly dampened by the approaching appointment time for occupational therapy. Although the resourceful occupational therapist amazes you with a knowledge of alternatives, there are the frustrating attempts to move food from the plate to your mouth, the difficulty in putting on your clothes and, worst of all, the embarrassment of relearning the necessities of the bathroom to deal with. With all that has happened, you just want to be left alone.

You wheel the chair down the hall as fast as possible. You know the occupational therapy aide will soon be at your door, eager to transport you to the therapy room. Finally, you find the solarium and manage to get the wheelchair through the door just in time. Ah, safety. You won't have to suffer the indignities of occupational therapy. Today, at least, your mind and body can have a reprieve from negativity.

Escape

When avoidance is impossible or impractical, then *escape* from threatening and negative situations can provide physical and psychological relief (Carson et al., 1988). The patient physically leaves the situation to escape the negativity and unpleasantness, and anxiety is reduced. Like avoidance, escape is a basic defense and provides immediate relief from frustration and *threats to self-esteem*. Self-esteem is a personal judgment of worth based on a self-ideal (Stuart, 2001a).

Patients with major neurogenic communication disorders may be unable to verbalize the need to escape a threatening situation. Often, there are only nonverbal indications that the patient needs to escape, indications such as agitation, fidgeting, and distraction. When these indications are present, the patient's wishes should be honored. Time out from demanding therapies and procedures should be provided for patients indicating escape needs. When it is necessary for patients to undergo procedures, the patient should be gradually exposed to them and provided with ample opportunities to escape the negativity. They should be able to pause threatening procedures and therapies until they can resolve the emotional issues.

You *Can* Run from Your Troubles

Sometimes you dread physical therapy. It hurts and forces you to deal with your defective arm. You cringe at the thought of being wheeled to the gym, where it seems everyone watches your every movement—or lack thereof. The sling holding your spastic arm is taken away, and strong, skilled hands pull, stretch, and try to increase its movement. Each movement sends flashes of pain down your back. Your stomach turns to a knot, and the anxiety and pain seem unbearable.

As the pain builds and the anxiety becomes too great, you try to find an escape. You utter a few words expressing your need to quit this painful and disturbing activity, but because of your communication disorder, the meaning is lost. The physical therapist seems oblivious or indifferent to your plight. You can't stand it.

Finally, you gesture the need to go to the bathroom. You make urgent noises and point to the handicapped rest room. At last the pain and the anxiety end, and you are wheeled to safety. You do everything you can to burn time and manage to spend the rest of the session in the rest room, free from the physical and psychological pain of your defective arm.

Ego Restriction

Avoidance leads to *ego restriction* (DeGroef & Heinemann, 1999), and it occurs in people who have severe feelings of inferiority. Ego restriction is a type of avoidance behavior used to protect the person from threats to self-esteem. The person using ego restriction refuses or abandons an activity because of pathological feelings of inferiority. He or she readily turns to another activity rather than risk the possibility of failure and the resulting loss of self-esteem (Mahl, 1971).

An early aphasiologist, Joseph Wepman, noted that in all instances of brain damage, there appears to be some reduction in the person's self-esteem. Self-esteem is derived from perceptions of self and the judgments of others (Stuart, 2001a). Although the amount of reduction in self-esteem and the extent of the brain injury do not have a one-to-one relationship, it appears to be a positive one. With the obvious exceptions of patients who have euphoria or denial, the more the brain injury, the more they appear to suffer from reductions in self-esteem. A patient's identity must change based on the new disability (Brumfitt, 1996).

Aware patients appreciate that they have suffered injury to their brains and, thus, are unlikely to have the abilities, thoughts, attitudes, and skills they once possessed. As a result, realistic, self-imposed narrowing of ego-boundaries is likely to occur and is a natural consequence of what has happened to them. For example, a teacher or attorney who recognizes that he or she cannot continue to teach or practice law because of the communication disorder is not acting defensively and irrationally. Their avoidance behaviors are natural, adaptive, and realistic, given the circumstances.

In ego restriction, however, the feelings of inferiority are unrealistic and maladaptive. Patients with neurogenic communication disorders employing ego restriction often have normal or near-normal abilities to succeed at the activities, but they refuse to engage in them. They fear that they will fail, and even the slightest likelihood of failure is so threatening that they unnecessarily limit their involvement. Sadly, because of their ego restriction, these patients never reach their rehabilitation potential.

When treating the patient who utilizes ego restriction, it is important to focus on his or her self-concept and self-esteem. Vocabulary exercises should focus first on egocentric names relating to body parts and clothing items, and gradually expand outward and away from the patient. Success at even minor tasks should be structured into the therapies, as the goal is to show the patient that he or she has the capability to succeed. When the patient fails, he or she should be shown that the failure was limited only to the task at hand and is not a general indication of inadequacy. Also, the patient should succeed more than he or she fails. What is most important is that the patient recognizes the implications of each successful performance and focuses on what he or she can accomplish, rather than focus on frustrations and failures.

Coffee Time

Few things in life gave you more pleasure than late-morning coffeebreaks. You loved gourmet coffee. The latte, espresso, mocha, or other elegant coffee was a delight for the senses. You eagerly anticipated the smell, sight, taste, and caffeine buzz the expensive coffees provided. Added to the delight of the coffee was the conversation. You and your friends would sit in the corner of the airy coffee shop, admiring the pastoral paintings, watching customers, enjoying the fresh air, and having fervent discussions ranging from politics to grandchildren. But the stroke changed all that.

Your speech has returned to near normal following weeks of rehabilitation. You can make the sounds of speech relatively clearly as long as you speak slowly and remember to exaggerate them. Oh sure, there is an abnormality to your speech, a sort of weird accent, but most people can understand you. You can make your thoughts known.

Your friends repeatedly invite you to return to the coffee shop. They sorely miss you. But you won't hear of it. You won't even entertain the thought of returning to the coffee shop. You have had brain damage. You know you will have trouble getting to and from the shop, ordering, and conversing. You won't risk the awful pangs of failure. You will stay home where it is safe and secure. No wheelchair ramps, no confused servers, no misunderstandings. Coffeebreaks are a thing of the past. They are now memories of better days, and you are perfectly content to let them go.

Fantasy

Fantasy is a symbolic way of meeting needs. It can be a form of escape through the process of daydreaming, which protects and supports the ego (Carson et al., 1988). Sometimes called autistic fantasy, the individual deals with emotional conflicts by using excessive daydreaming as a substitute for a more appropriate action (Burgess & Clements, 1998). There are a variety of fantasies, including occupational, athletic, financial, sexual, and social. During fantasy escapes, the person can retreat and withdraw into an imaginary world and bridge the gap between desire and reality (Carson et al., 1988). During this time, the person can act out emotionally significant roles in well-organized and often elaborate daydreams.

Fantasy also can be unconscious, fantasies embedded in the unconscious mind. Unconscious fantasy can influence a person's consciousness. This is particularly true of unconscious role scripts. For example, a person can act out an unconscious fantasy that he or she is impervious to danger, a rough and tough chance-taker. A patient with this type of script may take chances unnecessarily and have a cavalier attitude toward rehabilitation.

Fantasy, as a coping style and psychological defense, is desirable, mature, and adaptive for some patients with neurogenic communication disorders. Unobtainable wishes can be obtained, albeit symbolically, during fantasy escapes. Patients can also withdraw and retreat into imaginary worlds during fantasy escapes. Fantasies can provide patients with needed relief from the realities of a situation. Like all coping styles and psychological defenses, fantasy certainly can be maladaptive when it becomes a frequent and unnecessary substitute for reality.

Language is not necessary in order to use fantasy as an escape from unpleasantness. Patients with severe neurogenic communication disorders can use pure visual imagery during fantasy. Although patients with intact language can narrate elaborate fantasies, purely nonverbal fantasies can be created by patients without language.

Fetch

Another session of therapy. Sometimes you feel that you are on a "fast track" to rehabilitation that gives you very little time to appreciate your successes. Today, your mission is to compute numbers correctly. You find the right number of quarters in a dollar, count ten pennies to make a dime, add one column of numbers, and subtract this, that, and the other thing. You are not doing well with these numbers. Once, they were so easily computed, and now they seem to be monumental problems. A sense of failure overwhelms you. Whew! You stare at a door knob. For a few precious seconds, you see yourself in your backyard. Your golden retriever jumps to retrieve a well-thrown Frisbee. The freshly mown grass is green, flowers are blooming, and the white picket fence clearly marks the boundary of that wonderful place. You are normal once again. Again you throw the Frisbee and the dog grasps it in her teeth. But the words, ". . . would the loaf of bread cost?" brings you back to reality. As you, the dog, Frisbee, flowers, and grass dissolve in your mind, you now find yourself struggling to remember how many dimes are in a dollar. At the end of the session, the clinician will write in the chart that you have difficulty tracking and attending to tasks.

Other Coping Styles and Psychological Defenses

Although many authors have listed coping styles and psychological defenses relative to their maturity and positive adjustment value, the ones listed in this section are those that are more or less capable of being employed by patients with neurogenic communication disorders. The likelihood of them being used by aphasic patients was based on whether language was required for activation of the defenses. Consideration was also given to the tendency of aphasic patients to be concrete in their thinking patterns. The nature and adjustment value of these defenses were based on theories and research conducted by Carlat (1999), Chisholm (1993), Perry & Cooper (1987), Valiant (1977), Wolberg (1977), and others. Of particular value are the empirical studies of the psychological defense mechanisms relating them to global mental health: Perry & Cooper (1986), Valiant & Drake (1985), Jacobson, Beardslee, & Hauser (1986a; 1986b), Battista (1982), and Valiant (1977).

Suppression

The purpose of *suppression* is to keep negative thoughts, feelings, drives, and wishes out of consciousness. It is a voluntary exclusion of ideas and feelings from conscious attention. Negativity is eliminated by intentional avoidance of a particular pattern of thinking. Suppression differs from repression in that the latter is done involuntarily. The person who engages in suppression does so consciously and voluntarily (Stuart, 2001b). The patient with a neurogenic communication disorder may voluntarily suppress thoughts about the effects of it on job performance, rejection from family members, and the necessity for prolonged treatment. The negativity associated with loss of the integrity of the self also can be suppressed.

The aphasic patient may be impaired in the use of this defense depending upon the extent of the language deficit. The mechanics of suppression involve inner language. Negative internal monologues must be stopped and redirected to more pleasant topics. The verbal impotence observed with aphasia also impairs the patient's control of inner language. The result may be a limitation on the use of suppression as an adaptive, conscious attempt to cope with disturbing thoughts and resulting anxiety. Perseveration can also reduce the patient's ability to shift thought patterns (see Chapter 3). Once the negativity has begun, perseveration can perpetuate the preoccupation with the negative aspects of the disability. This problem can be addressed by an early start in treatment, with a positive attitude about success and outcomes. Support and encouragement by family and friends can also create a positive mental set about the disability.

Sublimation, Substitution, and Altruism

Sublimation, substitution, and *altruism* are categorized together because all three involve redirection of the negative to personally or socially acceptable attitudes or behaviors, and they are similar in nature. According to Stuart (2001b), sublimation is the acceptance of a socially approved substitute goal for a drive whose normal mode of expression is blocked. It is the channeling of personally unacceptable feelings or impulses into socially desirable behaviors. Sublimation differs from altruism in that the person employing the latter attempts to fulfill the needs of others as a way of fulfilling his or her own needs. Both can be considered mature attempts to cope with stressors. Both sublimation and altruism involve the individual engaging in unselfish methods of channeling negativity. Substitution closely resembles sublimation and altruism (a broad definition of *substitution of love objects* is not included in this discussion). Substitution is employed to reduce tension resulting from frustration and works by disguising motivations (Chisholm, 1993). An example of substitution is a person who feels unattractive, so he or she puts energy into sports (Chisholm, 1993).

Sublimation, substitution, and altruism are defenses capable of being employed by even patients suffering from severe neurogenic communication disorders. For example, a number of patients have written about their disability. Although people write books for many reasons, those on the recovery from illness are often written for altruistic reasons—to help others who have suffered similar plights. Even severely involved aphasic patients can sublimate, substitute, and be altruistic. Language is not required to engage in unselfish redirection of negative emotions and drives. Therapists are familiar with the patient who is eager to help others and assumes the role of nurturer in group therapy sessions. These defenses can range from writing elaborately about the trials and tribulations of recovery to assisting others with speech drills within the confines of their own disabilities.

Humor

Prazich (1985), a young dentist who suffered a CVA and a resulting communication disorder, wrote in his account of the recovery process, "After a stroke, it is very hard not be scared and feel sorry for yourself. A very good prescription for both of these feelings is laughter. As a result of losing control of my emotions, I discovered I felt really great inside after a good laugh. I knew this had some actual therapeutic value" (p. 29). With *humor*, an amusing aspect of a stressor or conflict is emphasized (Burgess & Clements, 1998). When it is used for the overt expression of feelings without personal discomfort, it is a mature defense (Carlat, 1999). Additionally, when humor is used as a mature defense, it must not be directed unpleasantly toward others.

The expression of humor, or the appreciation of it, is one of the highest language functions capable of humans. Humor is enjoyed by many individuals, but unfortunately, it is frequently beyond the range of the language-deprived individual. Although there are a variety of forms humor can take, such as slapstick, cartoons, monologues, and plays, many of them involve using language in unexpected ways. The humor defense requires a high degree of sensitivity to others and, with the exception of nonverbal, visually based humor, elaborate use of language.

Rationalization and Intellectualization

Rationalization functions to elevate self-esteem by disguising motivations and masking feelings. It is a conscious attempt by the ego to make unacceptable feelings and behaviors acceptable (Imboden & Urbaitis, 1978). Literally, rationalization means "making rational." *Intellectualization* and rationalization occasionally are used synonymously. However, they differ technically. Intellectualization is the tendency to place emotional conflicts on the intellectual level, thus removing the person from active emotional involvement. Abstract thinking is used to minimize disturbing feelings (Burgess & Clements, 1998).

Intellectualization is one form of rationalization. It is excessive reasoning used to avoid disturbing feelings (Stuart, 2001b). Rationalization includes the efforts of an individual to bring into a rational gestalt his or her conflicts and actions, and it is not only the making of excuses typically attributed to this defense (Walker, 1981).

It can be argued that rationalization is mature when it truthfully addresses the behavior or thought (Walker, 1981). The person justifies an act to remove himself or herself from the feelings associated with it. Of course, rationalization does not occur only with acts of commission; a person also can rationalize an act of omission. That is, he or she can attend to the acceptable reasons for neglecting or rejecting an act that should have been completed. The person ignores or denies unacceptable motivations for avoiding a necessary or morally desirable behavior. Rationalization is adaptive and productive when used truthfully, appropriately, and sparingly (Kolb, 1977). In excess, it can prevent emotional development and restrict a person's functioning. Excessive rationalization frequently occurs in patients with traumatic brain injury, and these patients often rationalize to their detriment. In these situations, rationalization should be discouraged.

Many aphasic patients are impaired in their ability to use rationalization and intellectualization. They are verbal defenses; the person primarily utilizes language to engage in them. Severely involved aphasic patients are unable to engage in the internal monologues necessary to rationalize or intellectualize conflicts, social disapproval, and unacceptable feelings and behaviors.

Some aphasic patients can profit from *externally imposed rationalization*. When the therapist provides truthful, accurate statements that reduce or eliminate negative feelings associated with an unavoidable act or omission, those patients suffering from reduced self-esteem may benefit from the rationalizations. The therapist provides the words, sentence structure, and intent for those patients incapable of it. For example, if a patient displays anxiety and indicates threats to self-esteem due to an inability to successfully perform as he or she once did naturally, the therapist provides rationalization for the unsuccessful performance. The therapist can say, "There is too much noise in this room, and besides, I presented material too rapidly." In this way, the clinician provides rationalization for the patient's unsuccessful performance. Of course, the patient's verbal receptive capabilities should be considered when using externally imposed rationalization. The externally imposed rationalizations should be adjusted to the patient's capabilities, truthful, and conducive to psychological self-protection. They are particularly useful for patients who are chronically frustrated and who have reduced self-esteem.

Repression

Repression is an automatic and involuntary regulation of unbearable ideas and impulses that are submerged into the unconscious realm (Chisholm, 1993). According to Carson, Butcher, and Coleman (1988), it is a defense mechanism in which threatening or painful thoughts and desires are excluded from consciousness, and it is an extremely important self-defense system. Repression, like denial, is one of the more common defense mechanisms. Many defenses are different manifestations of repression, and, in fact, repression is the common denominator of all defense mechanisms (Walker, 1981). In repression, events are detected and stored but are excluded from consciousness. When negativity arises, repression allows the ideas and impulses causing it to be excluded from the conscious realm. Carlat (1999) describes repression as "stuffing" the emotion out of conscious awareness.

Pre- and post-traumatic amnesia are associated with disruptions of neurochemicals. However, the memory deficits patients frequently suffer regarding events surrounding a cerebral insult may also be related to repression of psychologically painful experiences. According to Imboden and Urbaitis (1978), the patient may see illness as pure adversity. He or she may unconsciously interpret illness as a punishment for past sins, or there may be a vague feeling of guilt. "Often, however, the guilt-ridden patient who sees his illness as punishment fears that the fates have even more suffering in store for him. Such a person may have a prior history of constantly fearing that something bad is going to happen to him and reacts to physical illness as if the long-dreaded doomsday has arrived," write Imboden and Urbaitis (p. 30). Therefore, the patient prone to repression has the tendency to expel and withhold from conscious awareness events surrounding the catastrophic event. As noted above, several neurological explanations for memory deficits surrounding catastrophic health events also account for the presence of post-stroke or post-traumatic amnesias. Damage to the hippocampus and other brain structures has been shown to result in selective amnesias. However, repression of events surrounding a catastrophe can account for one of many factors associated with these forms of memory loss.

Repression is an unconscious process that helps the individual alleviate anxiety (Carson et al., 1988). The cerebral insult causing the neurogenic communication disorder may also permit previously repressed ideas or impulses to enter a patient's consciousness. For example, the brain-injured patient may no longer be able to keep repressed any painful thoughts of childhood. "The simmering, unresolved conflicts push to the surface; this is called the return of the repressed," says Chapman (1976, p. 61). Repression is a defense well within the range of the aphasic patient; language is not required to employ it. Unfortunately, conventional psychotherapy for repressional dysfunctions is beyond the range of severely involved aphasic patients to accrue significant benefit because these psychotherapies require communication.

Reaction Formation

According to Stuart (2001b), *reaction formation* is the substitution of attitudes and behaviors that are diametrically opposed to what one really feels or would like to do. It is the expression of an overt attitude or behavior directly opposite of underlying feelings, motives, and wishes (Burgess & Clements, 1998). It protects the individual by preventing painful or unacceptable attitudes from being expressed. Reaction formation can provide a permanent, effective defense against anxiety (Larson, 1984). Freud (1908) considered one manifestation of a reaction formation to be the general trait of orderliness and cleanliness. In some persons, it is used as a defense against the repressed desire to be messy and dirty. According to Mahl (1971), generosity can be a defense against unconscious stinginess. The chronic daredevil may behave in a careless manner to keep deep-seated fears repressed. Cheerfulness can be a reaction formation against underlying depression. One clue that reaction formation is present in a patient is the exaggeration of what is normally a socially desirable way of behaving (Mahl, 1971). "Too much, too often" are signs of reaction formations.

Reaction formation does not require language; it can be used effectively by all patients with neurogenic communication disorders. However, language is frequently required to show the nature of the reaction formation and to discover the source of the negative emotions. The ability to communicate plays an important role in the general formation and expression of a reaction formation. Exceptions to this would be obsessive cleanliness, orderliness, and overt nonverbal demonstrations of compassion. It is not postulated that all attempts by the patient for cleanliness and orderliness are reaction formations, nor that nonverbal acts of compassion and sacrifice are necessarily maladaptive efforts to reduce negative emotions. These acts can, however, signal an attempt to obtain relief from anxiety.

Displacement

Displacement involves the shift of emotion from a person or object to another, usually neutral or less dangerous and threatening, person or object (Stuart, 2001b). In displacement, a safer person or object is used as a substitute for that which actually arouses the feelings and impulses. According to Chisholm (1993), displacement helps the person disguise and redirect feelings. Hostile feelings for a supervisor at work can be displaced to a subordinate, and practical jokes can disguise feelings of hostility (Walker, 1981).

Displacement as an unconscious defense does not require language. It can be used by all patients with neurogenic communication disorders. Sometimes the therapist can be the "safe person" involved in displacement for both the patient and his or her family. The requirements for displacement to occur are met when it is recognized that the patient has suffered a significant, possibly irreversible, loss of communication abilities. Hostile feelings, anxiety, and fear and guilt about the circumstances or an emotionally charged situation can all be displaced to the therapist. Difficult, painful, expensive, and unpleasant medical treatments can generate negativity, and displacement is one way in which the patient, or his or her family, can reduce anxiety. Frequently, doctors are too threatening to confront, and the patient may choose nurses, therapists, and aides as less threatening people for the displaced anger and other negative emotions to be directed.

Dissociation

Dissociation is the separation and detachment of emotional significance from an idea or situation (Stuart, 2001a). This radical, desperate attempt at coping allows the person to remove painful feelings from conscious awareness. The individual dissociates rather than feel the pain (Carlat, 1999). Specifically, it is the separation of a group of mental or behavioral processes from the rest of the person's consciousness (Stuart, 2001b). Huelskoetter (1983) describes six types of dissociative reactions to severe anxiety: *amnesia, depersonalization, fainting, fugue states, somnambulism,* and *multiple personalities.*

Amnesia involves extensive but selective memory losses (Sarason and Sarason, 1993). Amnesia can be caused by organic or psychological factors, and when it occurs as a form of dissociation, it is the individual's attempt to separate himself or herself from information or experience. This separation relieves the anxiety and negative emotions associated with the experience or information.

Depersonalization is a sensation of isolation, unreality, and a feeling of loss of identity. The person's self-perception changes (Sarason & Sarason, 1993). The symptoms are transient, and the individual may say that a limb feels like it is unattached to the body. Depersonalization can occur during deep meditation and is called an "out-of-body" experience.

Fainting involves a complete and temporary loss of consciousness, and it serves to dissociate the person from reality. Fainting is related to a society's tolerance of it and in some cultures, it is tolerated more in women than men. Loss of consciousness (fainting) can occur in a patient with neurogenic communication disorders when he or she experiences a catastrophic reaction. Psychologically, the patient dissociates himself or herself from anxiety and associated negative emotions by losing consciousness.

Fugue state is the fourth dissociative reaction. A major change in personality occurs, with the patient becoming disoriented and confused. It is a massive dissociation of personality resulting in the tendency to seek physical escape.

TABLE 2   **Dissociations and Aphasic Patients**

Reaction	Observable	Reportable
Amnesia	No	Yes
Depersonalization	No	Yes
Fainting	Yes	No
Fugue state	Yes	Yes*
Somnambulism	Yes	No
Multiple Personality	No**	Yes

*The confusion may be reportable by higher-functioning patients
**Dramatic shifts in behavior may be observable

Somnambulism, or walking while asleep, is the fifth dissociative response and is common in children. In adults, it suggests pathological conflicts and is associated with dreaming physically active fantasies.

The last dissociative symptom is multiple personality. Multiple personality syndrome is rare and difficult to identify, unless the person is observed closely. The person lives two or more lives independently without awareness of the others. Recently, some authorities have questioned whether multiple personality disorders exist as a clinical entity.

The phenomenon of dissociation of the integrative functions of the personality in order to reduce or eliminate anxiety is within the range of even the most severely involved aphasic patient. Dissociation is a nonlanguage, unconscious phenomena. Of all the dissociation reactions, fainting is probably the most visible in the aphasic population and is associated with catastrophic reactions. For these patients, "vascular changes, irritability, evasiveness, or aggressiveness may precede or accompany the catastrophic reaction. An extreme catastrophic reaction may take the form of loss of consciousness" (Eisenson, 1984, pp. 187–188). Fugue state and somnambulism dissociations require intact physical abilities to perform, and many patients may be incapable of engaging in them. Psychogenic amnesia, depersonalization, and multiple personality require good communication abilities to effectively report and, as such, they may occur but remain undiscovered because of the patient's language deficits. Table 2 lists the dissociation reactions.

Undoing

According to Stuart (2001b), *undoing* is an act or communication that partially negates a previous one. It is the individual's attempt to deal with emotional conflicts by making amends, an attempt to undo and repair feelings or actions. A symbolic act to remove a previously conscious intolerable action or experience (Chisholm, 1993), undoing is an unconscious defense and an exaggeration of a normal process.

Mild to moderately involved aphasic patients and those with apraxia of speech and dysarthria are capable of engaging in undoing. For example, a patient under stress may reject the therapist, engage in profanity, or physically attempt to assault him or her, and later, verbally or nonverbally, the patient will attempt to undo the negative act. The patient may attempt to undo the negative acts by permitting therapy when he or she really does not want to be bothered or by completing workbook assignments instead of watching television. There also may be more overt attempts to negate the previous behaviors. Because of the symbolic nature of undoing and the necessity for patients to engage high levels of abstraction about the negative act and method of undoing it, this defense may be beyond the reach of severely involved aphasic patients.

Passive-Aggression

The *passive-aggressive* person indirectly expresses aggression toward others (Burgess & Clements, 1998). He or she indirectly expresses hostility through procrastination, delay, and other frustrating behaviors. The person requires approval and assurance, and the underlying hostility is masked by timidity and passivity (Kolb, 1977).

The passive-aggressive defense is unconscious and does not require language or symbolization. It is capable of being employed by all patients with neurogenic communication disorders. However, passive-aggression can be confused with memory deficits, lethargy, response-delay, and behavior problems frequently observed in frontal lobe syndrome (Tanner & Barnwell, 1994). Although patients can deal with stressors by the use of passive-aggression, brain injury and concomitantly occurring cognitive and behavioral deficits can cause a variety of organically imposed reactions that resemble passive-aggression.

Projection

According to Chisholm (1993), *projection* helps a person avoid awareness of his or her own undesirable wishes, emotions, and motivations. Stuart (2001b) notes that projection is an unconscious rejection of emotionally unacceptable thoughts or feelings and the attribution of them to someone else. In the extreme, the projection defense mechanism may result in delusions (Burgess & Clements, 1998). Chapman (1976) writes, "Freudian-psychoanalytic theory proposes that many delusions and hallucinations are projections of the individual's inner tumult and unacceptable urges onto the outside world" (p. 63). Projection allows the patient relief from guilt by blaming other people for one's own negative impulses (Walker, 1981).

Sometimes projection is used by the patient's family. Statements made by family, such as, "You don't spend enough time with my father!", "You don't put in as much effort with father as you do the other patients!", and "You don't seem to care whether he gets better or not!", can be manifestations of projection. Guilt is felt when a patient is placed in a long-term medical care facility. The patient's family may feel shame because of their inability or lack of desire to care for the patient. Projection also involves denial; a person must deny the negative emotions in himself or herself to be able to project them onto another. Of course, these statements also can be objective appraisals of the circumstances from the perspective of the family member of the patient.

Depending on the awareness of the patient, he or she also may use projection as a defense. For example, the patient's lack of motivation during rehabilitation can be projected onto the therapist. A patient's accusations of indifference on the part of the clinician can be manifestations of projection by the patient. Feelings of failure experienced by the patient can result in projecting negative assessments of the therapist's competency.

Regression

Regression is a retreat to a more secure and comfortable level of adjustment (Stuart, 2001b). It is the return to reaction patterns long since outgrown (Carson et al., 1988). Regression involves a reduction in the individual's anxiety by becoming more dependent.

There are patients who regress psychologically because of the stress associated with the neurogenic communication disorders. These patients, for example, may seek and find comfort in a dependent relationship. Regression to the immature role of a dependent child satisfies needs for security and comfort. Particularly during the early stages of recovery, the patient may benefit from this defense. The goal of rehabilitation, however, is to produce an independent, productive person, and the patient's regressive tendencies should be gradually discouraged and ultimately eliminated.

In summary, many coping styles and psychological defenses are used by people to protect themselves from unpleasantness. Some are adaptive, productive coping styles and defenses used to reduce anxiety and psychological distress. Other defenses and coping styles are radical, immature, neurotic, and maladaptive. Although the nature of coping styles and psychological defenses are the subject of continuing debate, the fact remains that

TABLE 3   Coping Styles and Psychological Defenses in Neurogenic Communication Disorders

Defense Mechanism	Use by Aphasic Patients
Avoidance	High
Escape	High
Ego Restriction	High
Fantasy	High
Suppression	Moderate
Sublimation, Substitution, Altruism	High
Humor	Moderate
Rationalization, Intellectualization	Low
Repression	High
Reaction Formation	High
Displacement	High
Dissociation	High
Undoing	Moderate
Passive Aggressive	High
Projection	High
Regression	High

people engage in them for psychological protection, and patients with neurogenic communication disorders are no exception. Table 3 lists some of the major coping style and defense mechanisms and the likelihood of their being used by aphasic patients.

CHAPTER

5

Neurogenic Communication Disorders and the Grief Response

I hold it true, whate'er befall,
I feel it, when I sorrow most,
'Tis better to have loved and lost
Than never to have loved at all.

—In Memoriam, Lord Alfred Tennyson

The only constant in life is change. The human experience, rich with discovery, acquisition, and growth, is also one of loss. Throughout their life spans, people share a common thread of acquisition and loss, and this experience with loss begins very early in life. Even for the infant, the gratification and satisfaction of breast feeding, and the closeness and intimacy with his or her mother that brings, is lost as age takes an early toll. Too often, the middle years bring loss of dreams and inevitable mid-life crises. Many people in middle age feel that they have lost the future or squandered the past. To the aged, loss is a frequent companion, with few new treasures to replace the ones lost. But without change, life becomes stagnant and static. Loss is a natural and predictable prerequisite to change. Loss is a shadow to life, a reality to recognize, understand, and accept.

Loss, and the feelings associated with it, can permeate the lives of people with neurogenic communication disorders. Patients with aphasia, apraxia of speech, and the dysarthrias may have a painful separation from loved ones, valued objects, and abilities. These communication disorders and frequently co-occurring physical limitations are the source of many real and symbolic losses. Often, they occur rapidly, with little time for people to prepare. Most aware patients with significant neurogenic communication disorders are overcome by loss and the human reaction to it: the grief response (Tanner, 1999; Tanner, 1997; Tanner, 1996; Tanner & Gerstenberger, 1996; Tanner & Barnwell, 1994; Tanner, 1987; Tanner, 1980).

61

Humans have various thresholds of awareness of loss. That which is a serious loss to one person may be a barely perceptible event to another. A loss that is traumatic to a teenager may be meaningless to a senior citizen. Certainly, not all occurrences of neurogenic communication disorders are of enough significance to merit the grief response. And, of course, some communication disorders are reversible. In mild neurogenic communication disorders, the patient may not feel that the losses are significant, or he or she may realistically perceive them to be temporary. In some patients, permanent separation from valued premorbid status does not occur.

There are factors related to brain injury that can reduce one's awareness of loss. For example, a patient in a coma does not have awareness of what has happened and, thus, does not experience the grief response. Patients in stupors do not have total awareness of their predicament. Consequently, they do not experience a complete sensation of loss. Some patients may have only partial awareness of the losses that can fluctuate over time. These patients can be more lucid at times, and during those periods of improved awareness, aspects of the grief response may be present.

Tangible and Symbolic Losses

When an individual loses an object, person, or aspect of self, he or she is separated from a valued aspect of his or her life. He or she tries either to overcome the losses or accept them. This process occurs for real, tangible aspects of the losses, and it also occurs for those aspects of life that have *symbolic* implications to the person.

Symbolic losses often involve a person's self-concept. Real, tangible losses can include people, abilities, and objects; they are discussed below. Symbolic aspects of the losses are related to the void and changes created in the person's self-concept. For example, a woman may lose her husband because of his death. The real, tangible loss results from the fact that he is no longer a part of her day-to-day life. His companionship, ideas, laughter, work products, and insights, are lost forever. The woman's husband and all of his exposure to her life have been taken away by death. The tangible reality is that she is permanently separated from a loved and valued person. She no longer can touch or speak to him.

The symbolic realities of the loss involve the void and changes the woman must make in her self-concept because of her husband's death. She is now a widow. Not only has the woman lost her husband, she also has lost a part of herself. One of the losses involves her role of wife and mate. Symbolically, the role may have supported her self-esteem. It may have provided a basis by which she defined important aspects of her life. More specifically, the woman's role of "wife to that particular husband" has been lost and never can be replaced. Even with a remarriage, she never can find a mate identical to the one lost, nor can she recapture the essence of time and experience shared with the deceased man. The real loss of her husband combines with the symbolic losses experienced by the woman in the grief response.

The Dimensions of Loss

There are three primary dimensions where patients with neuropathologies of speech and language feel grievous losses: *person*, *self*, and *object* (Tanner, 1997; Tanner & Gerstenberger, 1996; Tanner, 1996; Tanner & Gerstenberger, 1988). To a lesser extent, many patients also feel developmental loss and loss of security (Tanner, 1980). As discussed above, these dimensions include both tangible and symbolic aspects.

Except for the developmental dimension, the onset of loss in each category is usually rapid. Rapid loss occurs without warning, with little or no time to engage in preparatory grief. Before the loss, there may have been warnings that it was impending. However, the person may have been unaware of the signs because his or her attention was directed elsewhere.

Loss of Person

There are several ways one can experience unwanted separation from a valued person. Both real and symbolic loss of a person can occur through death, divorce, departure, and psychological separation. Only through death is the loss obviously permanent. In divorce, departure, and psychological separation, a person has the knowledge that the loss may be temporary; he or she may reconcile with the separated one. This knowledge can hamper the person's attempt to come to terms with the loss. Since there is a possibility that the person may be reunited with the lost one, acceptance of the loss is delayed or impaired.

Loss of person through departure occurs when one party simply leaves a marriage, intimate relationship, or living arrangement, with or without notice, and does not legally or formally finalize the separation. This voluntary separation tends to interfere with completion of the grief response because it lacks the finality of a legal decree and closure. A form of voluntary separation also occurs when a child leaves home for college, marriage, or a job. Although the separation is incomplete because the child may maintain aspects of the previous relationship, it involves loss because of the change in living arrangements and the resulting lack of intimacy. This loss of the intensity and stimulation of childrearing has been called the *empty nest syndrome*. Involuntary separation occurs when a party leaves a relationship through no fault or intent of his or her own. Kidnapping, induction into the military, and hospitalization are examples of involuntary separation.

A type of *psychological separation* occurs when one party in a relationship persistently avoids or refuses intimate contact with another. Psychological separation usually precedes physical separation through divorce or departure. When this happens in marriage, couples become disenchanted and avoid or refuse meaningful verbal or physical contact. The breakdown in communication further isolates the partners, and a spiral of negative emotions occurs because of the persistent lack of communication. This lack perpetuates the psychological separation. Although there may be some verbal and physical communication in psychological separation, it is superficial or meaningless. Communication becomes ritualistic. When a partner in the marriage or relationship recognizes the nature and extent of the psychological separation, the grief response can occur. Many individuals who have experienced a divorce report that the "death" of the marriage occurred months or even years before the legal decree.

Many individuals who suffer significant neurogenic communication disorders experience a psychological separation from loved ones. Families and friends of the patients also experience it. Although the patient may not physically lose his or her family members or friends, a psychological sense of separation can exist as a result of the communication disorders. Meaningful verbal communication is denied the participants in the relationship because of the neurogenic speech and language disorders. Particularly in aphasia, where the language disorder involves deficits in all modalities of communication, the patient and his or her loved ones are isolated psychologically from one another. This involuntary psychological separation often is compounded by actual physical separation when the patient is confined to a medical care facility. To further compound the separation, sensory deficits can reduce the extent to which physical contact can bridge the gap between the patient and his or her loved ones.

The role communication plays in developing and maintaining significant relationships cannot be understated. Before the aphasia, apraxia of speech, or dysarthria, the patient's relationships were created, nurtured, and maintained by communication. Problems that surfaced were addressed primarily through verbal means. Speech and language served as a means of sharing and venting emotions. Mutual problem-solving between the patient and his or her loved ones, especially in the areas of child-rearing and financial matters, was done verbally. Even for the patient who was characteristically quiet and reserved, speech and language were vital and necessary aspects to the development and maintenance of human relationships. The onset of the significant neurogenic communication disorder removes or impairs an important element of human bonding. Unfortunately, the stroke, head trauma, or disease that caused the communication disorder also creates significant levels of stress for the patient. The more severe the communication disorder, the more extensive the disruption of the patient's relationships. The grief response, in this case, results from the many changes that occur in interpersonal relationships. The relationship between the patient and his or her loved ones is altered significantly, and frequently irreversibly, by the neurogenic communication disorder. Although the patient has not lost his or her loved ones in a physical sense, he or she has lost the ability to communicate with them in a meaningful manner.

Loss of Self

Loss of self occurs when a person perceives that he or she no longer possesses some aspect of his or her physical or psychological integrity. There is also the loss of his or her status as a person in society (Brumfitt, 1996). *Loss of function*, one aspect of loss of self, occurs when an individual experiences an irreversible inability to perform as he or she once did normally. Loss of function may occur because of developmental changes, strokes and traumatic brain injuries, or degenerative diseases. The grief response occurs when the person realizes that he or she does not have the functional abilities of others.

The point at which a person becomes aware of the loss marks an important stage in his or her acceptance of the disability. This is true in all dimensions, but it is particularly important in loss of self. For example, the patient who has suffered a traumatic head injury and the resulting paralysis initially may not possess the perceptual and cognitive capabilities to understand the full extent of his or her impairments. However, as the patient's awareness returns, he or she will begin to appreciate what has been lost. Similarly, children with congenital disorders may never have been capable of unimpaired functioning but only come to appreciate this fact in childhood. The full realization that they are different and impaired in functioning may not occur until the child's perceptual skills, cognitive development, and experience permit it (see Figure 10).

Two types of loss of self are predominantly symbolic, and there are few, if any, tangible aspects to them. *Loss of time* and *loss of innocence* are primarily symbolic losses.

Loss of productive or meaningful use of time involves a person feeling that he or she has wasted part of life. A person may feel that his or her youth was misspent or that a period of life devoted to learning was not spent as effectively as it should have been. People who obtain college degrees in professions to which they find they are unsuited may feel that they have wasted an important aspect of their lives. Time devoted to an unsuccessful marriage may make a person feel that they have squandered "the best part of life." Wasting of time has few tangible aspects to it.

Loss of innocence, not merely in the sexual realm, is another primarily symbolic loss. When a person realizes that he or she no longer views the world with the innocence of a child, he or she may feel this as a serious loss. It is the loss of an innocent perspective on life. These predominantly symbolic losses are as irreversible and permanent as losses in other dimensions. It is impossible to recapture time squandered and innocence lost. Especially in aphasia, there can be a sense of loss of continuity with the past (Brumfitt, 1996).

The tangible loss of function involves the patient's specific disability. For example, a patient may be unable to walk. The referential loss of the ability to

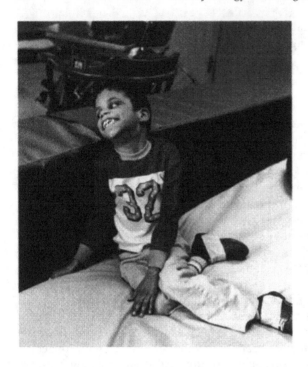

FIGURE 10   Full realization of loss of self may not occur until a child's perceptual skills, cognitive development, and experience permit it.

walk combines with the symbolic implications of the inability to come and go freely. To some people, the psychological implications of being unable to stand on one's own two feet can be more grievous than the physical disability.

The psychological and symbolic aspects of losing the ability to communicate are varied and many. To speak is to be potent. To be deprived of this fundamental ability reduces the individual to near-primitive levels of existence. Drives and wishes go unanswered. Expressions of emotions are reduced to the nonverbal mode, often leaving the listener confused. Life for the patient with severe neurogenic communication disorders can become an exercise in futility of expression—an awkward game of charades. Indeed, the symbolic effects of a neurogenic communication disorder can be profound and dramatically affect a person's quality of life.

Loss of Object

Loss of object can be very significant to a person. Valued objects include homes, jobs, money, automobiles, libraries, pets, sewing machines, gardens, recreational vehicles, etc. Loss in this dimension can include virtually any object or thing a person may have come to value. The objects of value are as varied as the people who value them. One person may place a high value on his or her home, another on a rock collection, and yet another on a vintage hot rod. Loss of the valued object has both real and symbolic implications for the person.

Loss of objects can encompass the intangible. People can be expected to experience grief over loss of culture, power, religion, and other beliefs. Frequently, loss of object is associated with symbolic loss. A person's valued objects, particularly intangible external ones, are assimilated into his or her self-concept. Loss of religious beliefs is an example of this type of loss of self. An individual who is subjected to one religious belief as a child and then loses it because of exposure to another religion can be expected to grieve over the perceived loss of the first religion. The loss involves both the objects and the rituals of the first religion, such as buildings, statues, and other physical representations of the church, and also ideas that are part of the religion's belief system. When a person no longer accepts the premise of the first religion, he or she loses both it and part of himself or herself.

People suffering from neurogenic communication disorders experience loss of objects because of the brain injury and resulting disability and also as a consequence of placement. For example, a patient can experience both tangible and symbolic loss of a motor home. He or she may appreciate the object as a well-designed and well-constructed machine, and it also may have symbolic value as a representation of the "golden years" of retirement. The neurogenic communication disorder and co-occurring physical disabilities can cause loss of this valued motor home because the patient can no longer use it. The grief response is a natural and expected reaction to the loss of the object. Unfortunately, because of the neurogenic communication disorder, the patient may be unable to express the nature of the emotional reaction to the loss.

Placement in a nursing home or long-term rehabilitation facility results in loss of objects for patients. Patients with a neurogenic communication disorder who are forced to move from their homes may experience a sense of loss over being separated from their garden, kitchen, pet, library, computer, or sewing machine. Many of these objects have symbolic value as well as practical utility. Lost objects create significant voids in the patient's life, and the communication disorder can prevent or impair his or her ability to report the nature of the feelings associated with the losses.

Developmental Loss

Developmental loss is perhaps the least identifiable of the losses experienced by the patient with a neurogenic communication disorder. However, the patient may indeed experience increased awareness of his or her developmental losses. In general, developmental loss is associated with the results of growth and aging. Developmental loss is usually gradual, but it can be brought rapidly into the consciousness of the patient by the onset of the communication disorder. Both young and old people lose in the developmental dimension. The younger individual loses valued aspects of life as more maturity and responsibility are required. Generally, the losses are not painful for infants and children because the things lost are easily and rapidly replaced by other aspects of life. Major loss during childhood is also a predisposing factor for adult depression (Stuart, 1998). The patient at the other end of the age continuum becomes more aware of the aging process and resulting developmental losses. The patient may feel suddenly that he or she is aging too fast and irrevocably. He or she can be expected to grieve over this process, natural though it is.

Loss of Security

The *loss of security* is the loss of the predictability of usual reinforcements. Security simply means that the individual knows what to expect. People experience insecurity because of factors they cannot control. The loss of predictability of usual rewards or punishments means that the patient does not know which attitudes, behaviors, and thoughts will result in external or internal rewards and which ones will result in punishments. The rules of the game have changed.

Some events clearly reduce the predictability of the usual rewards and punishments. One of the most significant events is the trauma associated with neurogenic communication disorders. Other events accompanied by high levels of insecurity include marriage, the birth of a child, a new job, moving to a new community, or divorce.

Patients with neurogenic communication disorders are prone to a lack of security as a direct result of both the brain damage and their awareness that life as they have known it is not likely to continue. In addition, there is the real threat of more devastating neurological impairments or death. Institutionalization itself creates insecurity for patients regarding new routines and therapy responsibilities. There is also the lack of security associated with financial responsibility for the necessary medical care. The patient knows that the services and institutionalization are very expensive and can drain the family's resources.

The Road to Acceptance

A *phase model* is useful in describing the grieving process (Boyd, 1998b). Grief is not one reaction. It is a complex progression of psychological adjustments to separation from something or someone of value. Before the 1970s, grief was viewed as depression primarily in response to death, and the way people coped with it was rarely studied, or even discussed for that matter. However, Elizabeth Kübler-Ross, a psychiatrist, proposed the first and most detailed outline of the grieving sequence in her landmark book, *On Death and Dying*. With this book, she brought the subject out into the open and detailed the process by which people accept unwanted change. Kübler-Ross was truly a pioneer in dealing with the subjects of death, dying, and grief.

Kübler-Ross is not without her critics. Some clinicians resist looking at grief as a phase model. They point out that not all people go through all the stages. They also note that many grieving people go back and forth between the stages. Some authorities believe that all depression is a result of a chemical imbalance in the brain, and loss only precipitates the abnormal biochemical emotional reaction. Actually, Kübler-Ross addressed many of these issues in her early writings, and her model is as viable today as it was in the 1970s. It has stood the test of time (see *On Death and Dying*).

With respect to irreversible neurogenic communication disorders, there are several reactions a person may have to loss. The patient with a significant irreversible neurogenic communication disorder, who has the cognitive and perceptual capabilities to be aware of it, will experience denial, frustration, depression, and acceptance. Of course, the patient must have valued that which was lost. The order of occurrence of the reactions may vary, and the time spent in a stage may be prolonged or brief. Losses in each dimension, tangible and symbolic, can result in the reactions. They may occur independently of one another or be present in such a way as to leave the person reacting to "loss in general"; the patient does not separate them but feels the sense of loss as an overwhelming emotion. Each reaction will be discussed separately in their usual order of occurrence.

Grieving Denial

Denial is usually the first stage in the grief response and is a reaction to unexpected, shocking news. It is a stage of shock and disbelief (Boyd, 1998b). Grieving denial can be prolonged or very brief. An example of this type of denial is the "I don't believe it" statement made by individuals who are initially confronted with a terminal illness or the death of a loved one. The basic defense adopted by the grieving person is disbelief and an inability to comprehend what has happened. It is generally accepted that denial is the initial stage of the grieving process, but denial may occur at any time. Some people may never use it, or it may be very brief.

Confrontation with the losses associated with neurogenic communication disorders may result in denial. It is an attempt by the patient to deal with the unexpected losses and to mobilize other, less radical defenses. The patient who successfully passes through the denial stage will move into stages of partial acceptance more easily.

As reported previously, denial is an aspect of many coping styles and psychological defenses, and it may be employed partially or completely (see Chapter 3). As such, denial, combined with other coping styles and defenses, may have four variations. With regard to neurogenic communication disorders, grieving denial can be *complete, partial, religious and mystical*, and *existential* (Tanner & Gerstenberger, 1996).

In complete denial, the patient does not acknowledge that he or she has a communication disorder. To the patient, problems occurring with communication are the result of the listener's inability or unwillingness to understand his or her perfectly normal speech. Not only does the patient completely deny his or her communication disorder, he or she projects the problem to the listener (see Chapter 4). In partial denial, the patient acknowledges that he or she has a communication disorder but denies the severity of it; he or she rationalizes that it is a minor, temporary problem. The denial is partial because the patient is aware, to some extent, of the communication disorder. Religious and mystical denial is employed by patients who believe their communication disorder will be removed by supernatural forces. These patients are usually passive in treatment programs and assume little, if any, accountability for the communication disorder. The locus of control in these patients is external. Patients with an internal locus of control accept the presence of the disorder and their responsibility in overcoming it. However, they deny the seriousness of it and believe that, though sheer will and determination, they can return to complete normalcy. This type of grieving denial is called *existential denial*.

Three factors influence the rate and ease with which the patient passes through grieving denial. The first factor is how much he or she is told about the disorder. If the patient perceives the extent of his or her illness but is told very little, successful mobilization of other defenses could be delayed. Another factor influencing adjustment in this stage is the time available for the patient to resolve denial. A patient may be aware of time constraints. If little time is available to the patient, as is seen often with the terminally ill, passage through this stage and other stages is frequently more rapid than might otherwise be expected. However, the opposite also may hold true.

The final factor that may affect the patient's ability to move through denial is his or her character before the onset of the communication disorder. Frequent use of denial throughout a person's life as a primary method of coping may suggest a strong learned behavior. The patient is likely to resort to this behavior as a means of coping with brain injury and subsequent communication disorders (Scott & Tanner, 1990). The past use of denial as a habitual method of coping increases the probability that denial will be a primary means of adjustment to the communication disorders and related losses.

Denial is a radical defense against loss. It takes a lot of psychological energy to deny reality. At best, denial allows time for a person to work into more acceptable thoughts and feelings. Denial is also a lower order defense. It does not require language to be employed and, thus, is available to aphasic patients. It serves as a buffer and provides the patient with time to mobilize less radical defenses to adjust to the losses. Grieving denial allows patients the opportunity to activate more adaptive responses to threats to physical and psychological integrity.

Grieving Frustration

Frustration results from the inability to obtain something wanted or to stop an unwanted event from happening. It is the result of a blocked goal. The amount of frustration is directly proportional to the drive for a goal or the strength of the desire to stop something. The frustration experienced by patients with aphasia, apraxia of speech, and the dysarthrias arises from two areas. First, patients are frustrated by their inability to communicate as they once did naturally and normally. There is a strong drive to communicate, and these neurogenic communication disorders impair or eliminate that innate ability. This inability to obtain a goal, *consummation of communication*, is acutely felt by patients with nonfluent aphasia, apraxia of speech, and many of the dysarthrias.

Second, the patient with a neurogenic communication disorder is frustrated by his or her inability to alter the course of events that led to the losses. Many *unalterable realities* are unwanted and frustrating. The patient may be frustrated by being confined to a nursing home or hospital. Required therapies, tests, and treatments can be frustrating. Understandably, a terminal patient would rather continue to live a healthy life than die. The frustration arises because of the patient's inability to alter significantly the course of unwanted events.

When denial can no longer be maintained, a frustrated person may experience *anger*. This level of adjustment is the result of the inability to maintain denial. Denial is replaced by anger, resentment, or even rage. On the positive side, anger can be considered partial acceptance of the loss that has occurred.

The grieving patient in this stage is difficult to treat, especially with regard to resentment. Resentment is remembered anger (Van Riper & Erickson, 1996). Although anger or resentment often is directed at health care professionals, it should not be considered a personal attack. Instead, it should be considered a random projection of frustration as a consequence of the circumstances. Anger is a natural and predictable stage in the patient's attempt to overcome the loss. Anger can also arise because of irritability due to depression (Carlat, 1999).

When the patient expresses anger, health care professionals may infer automatically a causal relationship between the patient's anger and their actions. It is important to remember that the accurate interpretation of anger in a communicatively disabled individual may be difficult. The patient may lack the abilities necessary to convey the nature of his or her frustration. Patients in the anger stage may feign indifference or show resentment. More overt signs of anger may be noticeable. Throwing food, bizarre behavior, and general lack of cooperation may be expressions of this stage of grief. The frustration and anger experienced by the patient may lead to depression (Chisholm, 1993). That is, *frustration leads to anger, and the inner direction of anger can cause depression.* Anger can be chronic and not related to the object or person to whom it is directed. Of course, health care professionals also may do or say things that make the patient angry. The important considerations are to look for the cause of anger and to allow it to be expressed.

Bargaining is also a reaction to frustration. The individual in this stage attempts to delay or reduce the effects of the loss. As with the previous stages, bargaining is normal, desirable, and helpful. The patient may bargain with God, family members, or even themselves. Bargaining also involves a degree of denial; the patient must deny the permanence of the disability. Most people, at some point in their lives, have attempted to offer good behavior in return for a reduction, postponement, or elimination of a negative event. Although bargaining tends to be unrealistic, it offers the patient more time to resolve the loss. However, extended periods of bargaining are counterproductive.

Bargaining also may occur with health care professionals. This stage is particularly relevant for those involved in rehabilitation. Patients in this bargaining stage can be highly motivated and enthusiastic about rehabilitation programs. However, unrealistic bargaining with the patient should not occur. It should be remembered that the ultimate goal of the grieving process is acceptance of the loss. Providing or supporting unrealistic ideas will stifle progress during this stage.

In patients with severe communication disorders, the bargain may be nonverbal, but higher functioning patients may verbally report the nature of the agreement. The form of the bargain may read as follows: "If I work hard and do everything you require of me, then, perhaps, I will get a return of all of my abilities." The bargain allows the patient to focus his or her attention on complete recovery rather than to experience an appropriate awareness of the disorder. Similar to denial, bargaining permits the patient to postpone complete awareness of the losses. It reduces frustration because it allows the patient to be unrealistic. Bargaining also reduces frustration because it permits the patient to relinquish the responsibility of the disorder. He or she is less frustrated, because it has been turned over to someone with superior powers to deal with the evils of the disorder.

Grieving Depression

Grieving depression sets in when all other attempts to overcome the loss have failed. The patient experiences a great sense of loss, and depression occurs when denial, anger and rage have run their course. The patient is no longer bargaining and acceptance is closer. Although grieving depression involves chemical changes in the brain, and can certainly go beyond a normal grief reaction, this type of depression is not psycho-organic. It is a reaction to loss and is independent of the damaged hemisphere and site of the lesion. Grieving depression is a natural and expected occurrence in aware people who have lost something of value.

As discussed previously, organic depression is associated usually with left hemisphere damage and typically seen in nonfluent aphasic patients with anterior perisylvian lesions. The amount of depression is related also to prolonged stress. Just as a child acts depressed or cranky when he or she is tired, prolonged stress in patients with neurogenic communication disorders is related to depression. Depression can also be a result of an internal direction of anger. Patients with neurogenic communication disorders are prone to this form of depression because of the problems they have with communicating and venting emotions.

The length of the grieving depression stage depends on the value the individual places on his or her loss. Losses that are less significant to the patient will produce less depression. In some patients, the depression lasts only a few days, but with others, it may last months. Some people who do not successfully pass through the stages of grief become fixated in depression. They never accept the loss and continue to grieve.

The patient who enters the depression stage of the grief response is aware of the losses. The griever recognizes the value of the losses and the fact that he or she is permanently separated from significant persons, functions, or objects. Additionally, the person's defenses no longer buffer or delay the reaction; depression results when the losses can no longer be defended against. Depression is a natural reaction to conscious awareness of significant losses.

The transition from bargaining to depression in the patient with neurogenic communication disorders is often accompanied by dramatic shifts in motivation. The bargaining patient usually is highly motivated in therapies because frustration is reduced by participating in the bargain. When the person reaches the depression stage, there is a reversal of motivation; apathy and lethargy set in. Physically, the depressed patient shows signs of despair. Some patients may be depressed and agitated, especially early on. Cognitively, the depressed patient does not attend well to tasks. During depression, the patient has difficulty maintaining attention to a task and often lacks enthusiasm and motivation.

Depression is a natural and predictable reaction to awareness of loss. When it is appropriate in magnitude and duration, it is considered a normal reaction. There are several factors to consider in determining the appropriate magnitude and duration of this stage of grieving. First, in normal reactive depression, the physical, cognitive, and emotional symptoms should be appropriate to the value of the losses. Second, the patient should not be at this stage longer than three months. After three months, even with the most significant of losses, the patient should have regular periods of normal affect. This is not to say that certain stimuli will not trigger episodes of depression. Brief episodes of depression can be triggered by stimuli for years following the loss of a very significant aspect of a person's life.

The third factor to consider when evaluating appropriateness and magnitude of depression is the patient's behavior. It is natural for the patient to want to avoid confrontation with the losses. It is also natural for the patient to desire an escape from the despair and suffering associated with this stage of grief. However, when the desire to avoid and escape from the realities of the losses include suicidal thoughts or actions, the depression is abnormal and should be reported immediately to the patient's attending physician. Reports of suicidal intentions are the main predictors that a patient may ultimately take his or her own life. These statements should not be ignored. Occasionally, some patients suffering from pathological reactions to loss will be depressed so severely that they will not have the energy to act on suicidal thoughts. Only when the depression lifts to a milder degree does the depressed patient find the energy to act on his or her suicidal tendencies. Similarly, chronic drug and alcohol abuse shows pathological reactions to loss and should be reported.

Depression should not be considered abnormal when it is associated with loss. Care should be taken not to project the attitude that depression is anything but normal. During this time, family members and friends may avoid the depressed patient. The spouse and other members of the family also may experience depression simultaneously with the patient. Understanding the process of grieving is beneficial not only to the patient but also to the family members and health care professionals (Keller, Tanner, Urbina, & Gerstenberger, 1989).

Acceptance and Resolution

Acceptance is the goal of the grieving process; it is the light at the end of the tunnel. Denial has run its course, and the patient's attempts to reduce frustration have proved unsuccessful. Realization of the loss and its implications has occurred. Usually, the acceptance stage is void of feeling. There is no attempt by the griever to resolve his or her fate. This stage is sometimes called *resolution*, and a person gradually experiences the return of well-being (Boyd, 1998b).

Early in acceptance, the resolution of the loss may be *partial* or *complete*. Partial acceptance is present when the patient is resolved to only part of his or her lot. A patient may accept hemiparalysis but remain unaccepting of aphasia. In the terminally ill patient, he or she may accept the eventual end of life but remain plagued by negative thoughts of leaving dependent children. Initially during acceptance, the patient may oscillate between it and previous reactions.

Resignation and acceptance are two different reactions to loss. Resignation implies that the patient tolerates his or her fate because there is nothing that can be done about it. Statements made by patients resigned to their predicament have the following theme: "I miss what I have lost, but there is nothing I can do about it, so I'll just have to put up with it." In resignation, the patient has not assimilated the loss into a psychological framework where he or she perceives it as a part of a greater, unalterable reality. Resignation is a result of denial, suppression, and repression rather than a product of working through the grief response (see Chapter 4). Accepting patients view their losses as neither good nor bad, just the way things are. The person is emotionally removed from them.

The accepting patient is also a good therapy candidate. If the acceptance is appropriate, that is the patient accepts the nature of the disability, he or she will continue to work at rehabilitation. In fact, the accepting patient may be even more realistically motivated toward rehabilitation than the bargaining one. The accepting patient can appreciate the likely results of his or her activities, whereas the bargaining patient may resist anything other than complete recovery and cling to unrealistic expectations. Accepting patients often will direct their energies more constructively because attention is now devoted to the rehabilitation process and not to grieving. He or she will not channel energy into psychological defenses against the loss.

Due to the patient's lack of emotion, family and friends may feel awkward and find it difficult to react to him or her. This also can be attributed to family members not having resolved their own feelings (Baker & Tanner, 1990). Patients with neurogenic communication disorders in this stage accept the situation but not necessarily their limitations. They continue to strive for improvement. Figure 11 illustrates the dimensions of loss and the stages of the grieving process.

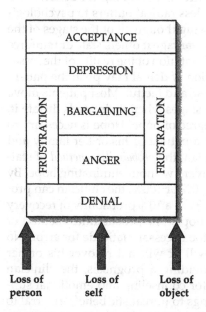

FIGURE 11   Stages of resolution of loss in neurogenic communication disorders.

Helping the Patient Through the Grieving Process

Several factors affect the normal grieving process, and many of them can be influenced by the clinician. Although there is little that can be done to prevent the losses that the patient experiences, thoughtful, caring clinicians can say and do things to help the patient reach acceptance of them. For patients who have experienced irreversible losses, the clinician's actions can be positive and assist in reducing the person's psychological pain. There are also actions and statements that can interrupt the process of accepting the disorder and its implications. The clinician should do all he or she can to produce an environment that is conducive to the patient rapidly moving through the grieving process. This may involve enlisting the assistance of family and friends in approaching the patient in the proper way. The patient's family members are important members of the rehabilitation team (Währborg, 1996). They should be aware of the way people reach acceptance of unwanted change (Tanner, 1999). Strategies used by the clinician to help the patient move through the grieving process are presented in the following pages.

Avoid Rewarding Denial

Rewarding denial can interrupt the course of the grieving process. Although helpful to a certain extent, denial is an extreme psychological defense and should be replaced as soon as possible by less radical buffers to psychological pain. Because of the importance of passing though all of the stages of the grieving process, it is not to the patient's advantage if others state or reinforce untruthful remarks. Of course, brutal confrontation of the reality of the losses also should be avoided. Brutal confrontation of denial may push the patient deeper into it. The goal is to be open, honest, and tactful. Most patients move naturally from denial to more productive stages when their needs dictate it.

All patients should be left with a degree of hope. Hope is necessary to mental health and to optimal recovery. If a patient or his or her family and friends ask for a prognosis from the clinician, the *probabilities method* of stating it can offer a realistic potential for recovery without eliminating hope. By avoiding the extreme percentages, such as 0% or 100%, the clinician can provide a prognosis without causing despair. Even a 10% probability of recovery offers something for which to strive and hope. The probabilities method of stating prognosis also gives the clinician the necessary latitude for error. No one can be 100% certain that a patient will or will not recover his or her speech and language abilities. After providing a prognosis, the clinician should allow patients and families time for counseling and emotional support. If the patient or his or her family clings to unrealistic beliefs, referral to a counselor, psychologist, or psychiatrist is warranted.

Avoid Contributing to Frustration

The patient with irreversible losses experiences frustration that causes anger and bargaining. The patient is frustrated by his or her attempts to overcome the loss and tries to defend against it. Frustration, and all manifestations of it, is a natural and expected aspect of the grief response.

The anger expressed by the frustrated patient takes many forms. Some patients display passive anger by refusing therapy or by isolating themselves. Severely involved patients can overtly express anger by throwing things, hitting others, or using obscene gestures. Less severely involved patients may call people ugly names or use profanity in an attempt to cope with the frustration. Many patients direct their anger inward. Patients with severe communication disorders are prone to inner direction of anger because they cannot verbally express themselves. Premorbidly, patients prone to inner direction of anger typically were verbal in their anger response.

Rarely should anger be punished or even discouraged. First, anger is an expression of feelings. As such, even in its raw forms, it is communication. For the severely involved patient, it may be one of the few feelings that can be expressed. Second, anger is a natural consequence of frustration and should be recognized as an important part of the grieving process. Acceptance of the patient and his or her predicament by family, friends, and health care professionals includes acceptance of the person's emotions. The patient's anger should be understood rather than reacted to by clinicians and family.

It is also important to understand that not all anger is a result of the patient's losses. All anger is not the result of grieving. Anger can be caused by insensitive family, friends, and health care professionals. Those around the patient should seek the cause of the anger and not assume automatically that it is a result of frustration associated with the losses. Carlat (1999) says, "The best way to diffuse hostility is to diagnose its cause and then target your intervention accordingly" (pg. 48).

Obviously, not all displays of anger are acceptable, constructive reactions by the patient. There are times when displays of anger should be discouraged. When the expression of anger is destructive to the patient, other persons, or a facility, intervention is required. This can be done in several ways.

First, the clinician should take care to stress that the anger is not being discouraged, but the negative manner in which the patient expresses it. Explaining this to a patient with severely impaired receptive abilities may be a challenge. (Anger is rare in patients with severe receptive deficits). Second, attempts should be made to redirect the patient's anger. For example, the patient should be provided with a harmless object that can be used for emotional ventilation. Also, it is not disastrous to a medical facility if a food tray is thrown to the floor by an angry patient. Neither is it disastrous if a chair is turned upside down because of the patient's frustration. Placed in the proper perspective, these acts are insignificant given the profound changes that have occurred within the patient. Allowing the patient to slap his or her hand on a table is an example of a relatively safe redirection of anger. If redirection of anger is impossible or impractical, the third approach involves restraints or punishment of destructive acts. Verbal punishment or withholding of pleasurable activities may be used in a program of behavior management. The least desirable alternative is the use of restraints, although sometimes they are necessary.

Bargaining, another manifestation of frustration, is a natural and necessary part of the grieving process. However, excessive bargaining can be problematic in itself. Hope is an essential element to acceptance but unrealistic hope should be avoided. As reported previously, patients with neurogenic communication disorders tend to be very motivated in therapies during the bargaining stage. This is especially true when bargaining occurs with health care professionals. The clinician can unintentionally provide false hope and perpetuate the unrealistic bargain because of what is said and not said. The clinician wants the patient to make maximum progress, and it is natural to avoid saying anything that will reduce the patient's motivation. It is difficult for the clinician to suggest that the patient's efforts in therapy probably will not result in complete recovery. There is the realistic fear that the patient will give up. Some patients do lose motivation when the bargain with the clinician is found to be unrealistic. Most do not. Although bargaining with the patient may produce positive short-term results, the long-term effects may interrupt the necessary grief work. Some persons fixate in bargaining and never reach an acceptance of loss. Patients in the bargaining stage often require more of themselves than is practical or desirable. In cases where complete recovery from neurogenic communication disorders is not probable, the clinician should counsel the patient to be realistic, yet optimistic.

A certain amount of frustration experienced by the grieving patient can be eliminated by the clinician. Sensitive therapists can structure the patient's activities to eliminate many unnecessary obstacles. As a rule in therapy, the patient should succeed more than he or she fails. The patient should be kept on a level of success that results in improvement. When a patient persistently fails at an activity, it is not his or her fault; it is an error in clinical judgment on the part of the therapist. The clinician needs to redefine the steps necessary to achieve the goals.

One of the first statements that should be made to the patient with a neurogenic communication disorder is: "You cannot force the word or utterance out." This needs to be communicated to the patient, by whatever means possible, early on. Easy trial-and-error exercises succeed at speech, whereas forcing speech results in increased frustration, anxiety, anger, and depression. When a patient continues to try to communicate something but is unsuccessful, the clinician should defuse the situation. This can be done by saying, "I don't understand now, we'll come back to it later." This acknowledges the importance of the patient's thought, but does not allow the frustration to continue.

Avoid Providing Secondary Gains

People empathize with the pain experienced by the bereaved. As a result, an individual in the grieving process may receive more attention, sympathy, and contact with others than he or she normally would receive. The support provided by friends and relatives is important to minimizing the pain experienced by the griever, and, as a rule, it should not be discouraged. Sometimes the attention, sympathy and contact provided by others, however, meet secondary needs in the griever. There can be *secondary gains* provided by the loss, and it may be difficult for the individual to give up the role of griever.

The following example illustrates the effects of secondary gains in a woman's attempt to obtain continued emotional support from family and friends, as well as her difficulty in relinquishing the role of griever.

> Nora, a 56-year-old female, was involved in an unhappy marriage to an alcoholic husband. Nora's spouse frequently physically abused her, especially when he was intoxicated. He also neglected her emotional needs. All displays of emotions by Nora were met with hostility by her husband. During a winter outing, Nora's only daughter was killed in a tragic snowmobile accident. The effects on Nora were devastating. After two years, the mere mention of Nora's deceased daughter resulted in severe and prolonged emotional outbursts. It was apparent to all concerned that Nora had not accepted her loss. The emotional pain, and Nora's dramatic reactions to the loss of her daughter, continued for years following the accident.

Nora's initial reactions to her daughter's death certainly were appropriate. She experienced a terrible loss. But the emotional reactions to the loss did not subside appreciably for years following her daughter's death, and secondary gains accounted for the prolonged grief response. When Nora would begin crying and wailing, her friends and relatives, even her husband, would attempt to calm and comfort her. This type of emotional support was lacking in her life and now met significant emotional needs. In fact, the only way Nora could display emotions was as the role of griever. Unfortunately, these secondary gains prolonged her grief and pain.

Lonely patients, especially those confined to a nursing home, may receive secondary gains from prolonged grieving. They receive attention from clinicians on a regular basis, and unfortunately for some patients, these clinicians may be the only outside visitors they get. Sometimes, this contact with a kind, caring person can result in an interruption of the grieving process, and less progress is made in speech and language recovery than otherwise would be possible because of secondary gains. Clinicians should be careful not to create emotional dependency.

Avoid Drugs that Are Heavily Sedating

Most physicians appreciate information from therapists about the nature and dosages of medications provided to rehabilitation patients. Many physicians recognize the value of the close relationship and contact between the patient and therapist when assessing the effects of medication on the patient, especially in the psychological realm.

For the grieving patient, tranquilizers, sedatives, alcohol, and similar drugs should be avoided during the acute stages of the grieving process. Awareness of the loss is an important step toward eventual acceptance of it. These drugs can interfere with the awareness phase and do not eliminate the emotional pain associated with loss, they only postpone it. Certainly, there are cases where medication is advisable and beneficial, but using heavily sedating drugs to eliminate the grieving process is contraindicated. Medications cannot resolve a crisis, but psychopharmacologic agents can help reduce its emotional intensity (Boyd, 1998b). They are beneficial when used temporarily or when other options are not available.

Emotional lability and grieving depression share common symptoms. Frequent and intense emotional outbursts may be indicative of persistent emotional lability (see Chapter 3) or unresolved loss and fixation in depression. With both disorders, an effective treatment may be mood-elevating medications. Even in these cases, however, the medications should be periodically reduced or removed in order to decide if the patient can regain emotional inhibition or reach an acceptance of the losses without them.

Avoid Interruption of Private Grief

Privacy is hard to come by in many medical care facilities. Most hospitals and nursing homes place two or more patients in a room. Additionally, some facilities either inundate the person with activities or totally neglect him or her. Both extremes should be avoided. The grieving patient should be provided with regular times and places so that he or she can be alone. The patient needs time and opportunity to become aware of the losses and to work through them.

Sometimes, friends and relatives suggest that the person become immersed in work or a hobby. The assumption is that the patient can attend to other activities and, thus, forego the pain associated with the losses. During the later stages of the grieving process, these suggestions may be necessary and helpful, especially if the patient experiences fixations in any stage of the grief reaction. Overindulgence in work or a hobby during the early stages of the grief reaction, however, may be counterproductive. The patient may be avoiding confrontation of the loss. Unhealthy early distractions can include moving to a new community or a new job, or the demands of an intensive rehabilitation program.

Permit the Patient Control

The psychological pain felt by a patient with a neurogenic communication disorder during the grieving process is partially due to his or her impotency in altering the course of unwanted events that led to the losses. The feeling of helplessness that accompanies grieving can be reduced by allowing the patient to control certain aspects of his or her life. Lack of control in the patient's life contributes to his or her frustration and anxiety about the loss or losses. The more control the patient has over his or her life, the less frustration he or she will experience.

In many medical care facilities, the staff dictates when the patient can engage in many day-to-day activities. The institution's routine reflects the staff's—not the patient's—needs. The result is that many day-to-day activities of the institution are outside the patient's control. The patient must wake at the times demanded by the staff, eat when the tray arrives, and go to therapy when the schedule dictates. Even visiting hours are set by the facility. There is little the patient can do to control even the minor aspects of his or her life. The dehumanizing effects of rigidly adhering to others' schedules combine with the fact that the patient is blocked in his or her efforts to stop the course of the losses, so it is no wonder that many patients react with bargaining, rage, and depression.

Patients with communication disorders lack the level of control that those with intact powers of speech and language possess. A verbal person can demand his or her rights, request privileges, and resist impositions. A verbal person often will get his or her way; indeed, "the squeaky wheel gets the grease." But the patient with neurogenic communication disorders often is at a distinct disadvantage. Too often, the medical staff neglects to discuss preferences regarding facility routines with the speech and language disordered patient.

The health care professional can be instrumental in providing the patient with control. He or she also can advocate for the patient with other members of the staff to create conditions where basic decisions can be made by the patient. Many decisions made *for* the communication disordered patient can be made *by* him or her. It is not difficult to create an environment where the patient can make most of the decisions about his or her day-to-day activities. For example, the patient can be allowed to decide which room to use for therapy or if therapy should be provided on a particular day. Higher functioning patients can decide what activities to emphasize in therapy and when to take breaks. The same principles can be applied to other therapies and nursing procedures. Medical care routines should reflect the patient's needs and not those of the institution.

Provide the Patient with Perspective

During the acute stages of the grieving process, the patient may feel that there will never be an end to the emotional pain over the losses. The patient may feel caught in a vicious cycle of loss and grief. During this time, the clinician can be of immense help to the bereaved by providing perspective regarding the eventual acceptance of the losses and the reduction of sorrow that accompanies acceptance. By placing the loss in perspective, the clinician allows the patient to see the light at the end of the painful grieving tunnel.

Perspective may be provided to the patient by telling him or her about the grieving process. The clinician should explain that the sorrow and pain will end; the process the patient is going through is one of healing. Counseling should be employed to help the patient realize the finite nature of grieving and become aware, on a personal level, that the pain and sorrow will subside. It can be comforting to a grieving person to have someone explain that there will be an end to the sorrow and that life again will have pleasures and joys in it. However, communicating this to a patient with severe receptive language deficits is challenging. One way of doing this may be to provide examples of patients with severe aphasia who, by their manner, appear to be well-adjusted and accepting of their disability.

Acknowledge the Reality of the Loss

It is natural for the patient's family, friends, and health care professionals to want to avoid discussion of what has been lost. Some people believe that by changing the topic of conversation they are helping the griever. But when family, friends, and health care professionals avoid discussing the losses, they deprive the patient of necessary and productive expressions of grief. To grieve properly, the patient must become aware of the losses and acknowledge the reality of them. In this process, the clinician can serve a very important function.

Unless the clinician has known the patient in the past, he or she is considered a *detached observer* concerning the losses. As a result, the patient may not feel the need to maintain a role and be inhibited in his or her emotional expressions when communicating with the clinician. For example, the patient with a neurogenic communication disorder may also be a husband, father, grandfather, or friend, and because of these different roles, he may feel the responsibility to act in a particular way. The patient may not feel comfortable expressing fear to his wife or children. Anger may not be expressed uninhibitedly to his or her friends. The clinician, however, is devoid of many sensitive roles, and, as such, the patient may feel less inhibited expressing personal and complex emotions. The patient may be more open to a detached observer than he or she would be to loved ones.

When confronted with the grieving patient, some individuals feel the need to explain, defend, or rationalize the losses, and this is not necessarily disruptive to the process of reaching acceptance. Many bereaved individuals welcome advice, suggestions, or philosophies of life presented in this way. However, silence often is therapeutic, and it may be welcomed by the patient. He or she may just need someone who will listen (see Figure 12).

Sometimes, people who encourage the patient to express the meaning of the losses will feel that a statement must be made that will "make it all right." There are no expressions that will permanently eliminate the pain felt by the bereaved. These attempts, however well-intentioned, are rarely appreciated by the patient and are often perceived as attempts to negate the losses or his or her feelings about them. It is also possible that what someone

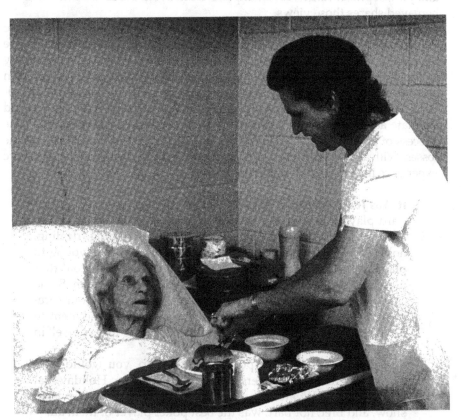

FIGURE 12   Listening is an important part of facilitating the grieving process.

DO	DON'T
1. Permit the patient control	1. Reward denial
2. Provide the patient with a realistic perspective	2. Contribute to frustration
	3. Bargain with the patient
3. Acknowledge the reality of the losses	4. Provide secondary gains
	5. Provide early distraction
4. Listen	6. Interrupt private grief

FIGURE 13   Facilitating the grieving process in neurogenic communication disorders.

intends to be a positive statement may be perceived as inappropriate by the patient. His or her beliefs may be different. People who have strong religious and philosophical values, for example, should avoid the assumption that the bereaved shares those views.

It is part of the clinician's responsibility to do all he or she can to facilitate the grieving process in patients with neurogenic communication disorders (see Figure 13). Helping a patient accept loss is as much of a clinical responsibility as the therapies. No matter what the dimension of the loss is, the clinician should regard the patient as being in a period of significant change and transition. The goals of rehabilitation include facilitation of the grieving process and ultimate acceptance of the losses by the patient and his or her family. The process of grieving helps the bereaved appreciate the true significance of the losses. With appropriate intervention, resolution of the losses can be a positive experience in growth and transformation.

It Was Just a Matter of Time

Card playing has always been therapeutic for you. From Gin to Solitaire, there is something calming about shuffling, dealing, holding, and handling cards. Even when you were too young to play serious card games, you would lie next to that big old fireplace on cold winter nights and make houses out of them. Some cardhouses would have two or three stories and only your carelessness, or your big brother's meanness, would cause them to tumble to the carpet. You have always been able to lose yourself in Jacks, Kings, deuces, and eights.

You especially love poker. Growing up, you would read about the great card players of the Old West: Doc Holiday, Bat Masterson, and Wyatt Earp. *Maverick* was your favorite television show, and Bret, not Bart, was the best poker player of them all.

In college, the weekly poker game was your favorite outlet and, you might modestly say, a good source of income. Early on, you learned to keep your beer consumption to a minimum and let the others make foolish, costly mistakes, like drawing to an inside straight. For years before entering this nursing home, you would have weekly poker games with your friends from work. Each player would bring chips, nuts, crackers, and beer. Ah, the smell of a cigar still returns you to those wonderful evenings of boasts, bluffs, and bets. Even now, sitting at this cardtable with quad canes, walkers, and wheelchairs parked next to it, you still love a good game of poker. Lately, though, it seems the stakes have been getting higher.

Your stroke happened eight months ago. It was the darndest thing. You had just gotten up and were opening a new can of coffee when your right hand wouldn't twist the can opener. Then, in a flash, your whole right side gave way. Thank goodness, your fall to the floor alerted Terry. You don't remember the ambulance ride to the hospital or the hours spent in the emergency ward. Nor do you remember the worried looks on your children's faces or the loving hugs of your grandchildren. For weeks, you were in an oxygen-starved neverworld, partially knowing what had happened and partially, wonderfully, oblivious to the terrible event that had taken so much from you.

During your stint in the rehabilitation unit, you started having flashes of awareness of all that had been taken by the stroke. You couldn't walk, even if you could get out of bed by yourself. Eating was done with the assistance of a nurse's aide. And, oh, the indignities of being unable to get to and from the toilet without help. Stuck in the hospital, you were separated from your home, car, kitchen, and weekly poker nights. You missed the security of routines, your dog, Rosie, and your evening walks with the crisp crunching snow beneath your shoes. You sorely missed the little things, those nightly walks, your dog, and the white vapor rising from your lips.

But the stroke has taken far more than your balance, poker nights, and walks. It has taken your loved ones. Oh sure, Terry, the kids, and grandchildren are still physically there. They were not taken from you by death. But, because you can't communicate, your life with them has been reduced to the basics. You want to talk to them about the big issues—the costs, the options, the future—but the bridge of communication has collapsed. You reach out for meaning in those relationships but are thwarted by verbal impotence.

Your life has changed, and as time marches on, you realize many of the changes are permanent. Even though you regained some of the abilities to walk and talk, the unwanted realities of life after stroke persist. There is now a great distance between you and the people and things you so cherished. Like losing the big pot in poker, the stroke has taken your life's winnings.

The burden of losing so much, so fast, is buffeted by your mind's defenses. Just beyond the senses, your mind blocks the painful realities of loss. There are minutes and even hours where you are oblivious of your plight. In denial, you find relief from the pain of loss. You have brief periods of respite where the sad reality of loss is gone. You hide in the corner of denial, shielded from the all-encompassing pain of loss. Denial is like a protective door allowing reality to enter gradually and slowly, when you deem the time is right.

The frustration of your predicament causes anger to rear its ugly head. You have been dealt a bad hand, and there are no more draws. You would like to change the reality of the situation, but on a deeper level, you know that is impossible. It angers you that you cannot do the things that once came easily. It angers you that your loved ones are unreachable, like some large cavern separates you. It angers you that Rosie walks alone at night.

Perhaps, you bargain, if you work hard in therapy or find a "miracle" therapist, doctor, or drug, your life will return to normal. You would pray for help, offer a vice for a reprieve from these losses, but even prayer has been taken by the communication disorder. The intimate words shared between you and God have been taken by the devil stroke.

You finally give up trying to overcome the losses. It's futile. The denial no longer buffers the pain, the anger serves no purpose, and there are no bargains to be struck. The cards have all been turned over, and you have lost the hand. The pot of life's valuables no longer belongs to you. Ironically, you feel the full value of that which was lost as the depression overwhelms you.

The depression you feel is not the result of chemicals gone awry in your brain. The depression you feel is grief. Humans are no strangers to it; it has been in the cards since the beginning. But that knowledge doesn't help reduce your pain, your cross to bear. You fall into lethargy and sadness, preoccupied with thoughts of those beloved people, things, and abilities that have been taken from you. Thoughts of death, dying, and loss saturate your heart and mind. You wonder about the meaning of it all.

The pain of loss gradually subsides. One afternoon, you realize that hours have gone by without the pain of grief. Hours of calm acceptance gradually become days and weeks. You soon realize that acceptance is not the same as resignation. In resignation, you only tolerate what has been taken from you. In acceptance, you understand the losses in the scheme of things, a scheme of which you are a part. Loss was always in the cards, and there would be no excitement in poker without it. You know that there would never be the joy of a royal flush without the sorrow of drawing 2, 3, 4, 5, 7. You find yourself basking in the pleasure of knowing what you had, rather than saddened by the passing of it.

The steps in reaching acceptance were not smooth nor did you escape backslide. Some steps were brief and almost skipped, while others made your feet of clay. Your difficult journey to acceptance was helped by your friends and loved ones. It seems that people just naturally know what to do. After all, loss has been around forever and so too has the compassionate human spirit.

As you watch the cards being dealt for the last hand of the night, you realize that your life has not really been a gamble. Poker is not a metaphor for life. In poker, the outcome is unknown and determined by skill, luck, and chance. In life, loving and losing were determined long before your consciousness arose from matter and energy. Life is not a game of Texas Hold-Em, and nothing was ever more certain than love and loss. It was all a matter of that persistent illusion called "time."

PART TWO

On Coping With Neurogenic Communication Disorders: Original Short Stories

"Life is a handful of short stories, pretending to be a novel"
—Anon.

"Cautious Clyde's Descent into Darkness"

Clyde felt more secure landing at Spring Valley Airport than at any other tower-operated airstrip in the state. It wasn't because Spring Valley was controlled better than other airports of its size, it was because the small airport had little traffic, and the calm winds flowed north to south, the same way runway "one eight five" coursed. The surrounding pine-covered mountains left little to the demands of navigation. A pilot had to be blind to miss Spring Valley. The Sawtooth mountain range was to the north, Lake Mary to the east, and to the west was the burnt ridge. Lately, the green was returning to the ridge; golden wildflowers could be seen, and the underbrush was gaining a foothold on the steep, rocky slopes. The residents of Spring Valley never discussed the burnt ridge, they seemed to accept the blackened expanse of the fire's wrath with the same tolerance they displayed for the cold dry winters of the Rockies.

Clyde considered himself a good pilot, as do all pilots, but Clyde's record supported his belief. He'd never as much as scratched a wing of an airplane, never dented a fuselage. Of course, few living pilots have scratched a wing of an airplane or dented a fuselage. In aviation, minor mishaps are rare, and somehow the word "mishap" is a misnomer when labeling accidents in midair. You don't have mishaps, you have disasters. Clyde was sometimes too cautious, but he was a cautious pilot nonetheless. This flight was no exception. Rather than contacting the tower when he reached the highest peak of the Sawtooth range, which was about five miles from the airstrip, Clyde would insist on contacting Spring Valley Tower a good ten miles from the airport traffic area. FAA rules were as clear as the bureaucrats could make them, and five miles was the minimum contact distance for incoming flights. Clyde was cautious all right; if five miles was safe, ten miles was safer.

"Spring Valley Tower, Cessna three four four five niner, ten miles north, inbound for landing," Clyde hailed in his most relaxed pilot's voice. He could barely see the top of the tower from his ten-mile vantage point. The brown log-constructed building's paved runway was a welcome sight to many a lost pilot. The joy of finding the airport from the green expanse of pine trees was directly proportional to the amount of fuel remaining in the airplane's fuel tanks.

A few seconds later, the tower responded to his hail. "Cessna three four four five niner, Spring Valley Tower. Left traffic, runway one eight five, winds one seven zero at five, gusts to fifteen, altimeter two zero zero eight. Report downwind. Your traffic is a Piper on final."

Clyde adjusted his dark glasses as he acknowledged the landing instructions into the microphone attached to the left muff of the Sony headset: "Cessna four five niner."

Eight hundred hours. Eight hundred and seventy-two hours to be exact. That was the time Clyde had logged in single-engine land aircraft. Those hours made responding to airport instructions as second-nature as obeying the only traffic signal in downtown Spring Valley. Nicole, the tower operator and a friend of twenty years, simply wanted this blue Cessna, with the white markings N34459 and the colorful hand-painted eagle on each side of the tail, to turn parallel to the runway and to keep a southerly heading. As per Nicole's request, Clyde contacted the tower when the parallel turn had been completed.

Gusts of wind up to fifteen knots were not a problem, especially when they coursed from the south. Crosswinds were occasionally a problem, but not here and not today. It would be another safe landing. At least that was what Clyde thought.

Clyde descended to 1,000 feet above the Ponderosa pines. He reduced the power to 2,000 RPMs, and ten degrees of flaps slowed the decent. He heard a reduction in noise when he cut the power, and the quiet reminded Clyde to lower the nose of the plane. "Keep your nose down and your speed up", echoed the words of his first flight instructor.

On the next turn, the plane slowed even more as Clyde added another ten degrees of flaps. Once again, he lowered the nose and pushed the hand-held throttle to increase his speed, then gave the tower a final notification of his intentions: "Cessna three four four five niner on final." A few seconds later, he heard Nicole's professional voice clear him for landing as he added the final adjustment of the plane's flaps.

Flying is boring. Well, a lot of the time it is boring. Once the airplane is in the air and vectored to its destination, there is little for the pilot to do. An adjustment here and there, and the plane automatically and obediently cuts the air to its destination. Takeoff is fun. There is that pleasant sensation as the airplane lifts from the confines of the runway to the freedom of the sky. But landing the airplane is the biggest challenge of all. So much to do, so much to know, so many things that can go wrong. The landing strip seems so small and approaches too fast. Worst of all, you are low, slow, and heavy, giving little time and few options if something goes wrong. And today, for Clyde, something went terribly wrong.

About a football field from touchdown, a gust of wind blew his Cessna to the ground. There was no warning, no advance notice. The down gust of wind simply caused the plane to drop like a rock to the pavement below. Clyde had little time to react. As per training and experience, he applied full throttle to gain speed. But it was too little, too late, and he was too low to the ground.

Just before the Cessna hit the ground, Clyde pulled back on the yoke and braced himself. These were reflex reactions, as was his denial. He didn't believe what was happening; he knew airplane crashes always happened to the other guy. But this time, he was the other guy. On impact, the right wheel strut broke, causing the airplane to tip to the right, while the nose and wing of the airplane dug into the pavement. The propeller bent and abruptly stopped. Clyde felt the seat belt and shoulder harness cut into his waist and shoulders as he was thrown forward. Then the blue Cessna with the white markings N34459, and the colorful hand-painted eagle on each side of the tail, simply flipped over and slid to a halt on the asphalt.

The impact caused the fuselage to crush like paper. The engine of the airplane broke from its mounts and pushed back into the cockpit and, in doing so, broke both of Clyde's legs. The top of the cabin of the airplane collapsed on impact, and Clyde's head slammed into the instrument panel. The plane skidded to a halt, sparks flying and smoke rising. Clyde's last thought was of the high test fuel in the wing tanks of the airplane and the explosion he hoped was not inevitable.

Nicole watched Clyde's final descent to the airport. She never tired of the grace and beauty of an airplane, no matter how small, in its careful, controlled transformation from an air machine to a ground one. She thought of Clyde carefully and skillfully controlling the flying machine. When she saw the Cessna hit the pavement, flip, and skid, for an instant, she did not believe her eyes. When the disaster finally registered in her mind, she automatically hit the large red button on her control panel, which sounded the emergency alert. She had never pushed the red button for real, outside the monthly routine tests, and it surprised her how loud the siren was, and how it disrupted the morning calm.

The "wherrrrr, wherrrrr, wherrrrr" of the emergency siren sent two red trucks to the crumpled Cessna. The larger red truck sprayed chemicals on the smoldering airplane. A man dressed in a bright yellow spacesuit jumped from the smaller truck and ran to the pilot's aid. Clyde was hanging from his seat belt and shoulder harness, blood flowing from his head. He was unstrapped and pulled a safe distance from the smoking wreck. Soon, an ambulance from Spring Valley Hospital arrived, and attendants secured him to a gurney and rushed Clyde to the only hospital in the county.

Eventually, the Cessna was completely drenched in chemicals. Thanks to God, luck, or the aeronautical engineers at the Cessna plant, the fuel in the wing tanks did not explode. Other airplanes were diverted to nearby airports, and the ones short of fuel were allowed to land on the narrow taxi strip.

As regulations required, Nicole notified the National Transportation Safety Board (NTSB), and an investigator was sent to determine the cause of the crash. Somehow, determining the cause of the crash seemed to bring closure to it. Of course, the cause would be "pilot error." It seemed it was always the pilot's fault. If the wings of an airplane were struck by lightning and blown to bits, it would be pilot error. In the view of the NTSB, a non-erroring pilot would dodge the lightning. Ultimately, it was determined that Clyde, cautious Clyde, was too slow and too low for the weather conditions. The downgust of wind and the crash could have been avoided by a better pilot, a safer one.

Clyde did not register the months that passed since the crash of the Cessna. The passage of time for a person in a coma has often been compared to sleeping. It is not. The biggest difference between sleeping and a coma is that a sleeping person can be awakened. And people in a coma also sleep. But nothing could awaken Clyde during those months. Not pain, not hunger, not the shouted words from his family and his friend, Nicole. For Clyde, those months were full of darkness. He might as well have been in oblivion. There was no awareness of himself or the expensive hospital room that had become his home. There was no passage of time for Clyde. From the last frightening images of the airplane crash to the sounds and blurry images he experienced months later, Clyde was in limbo. It was like he was on automatic pilot.

The formal diagnosis on Clyde's chart was "traumatic brain injury—closed." This simply meant that during the crash of the Cessna, his head slammed into the instrument panel, damaging and killing brain cells. The massive amount of blood covering him and the cockpit of the airplane came from his head, but only the surface areas. There was no penetration into his brain. Even minor head wounds bleed profusely. Initially, there was a buildup of blood inside his brain. The broken blood vessels spilled their contents into his head, and with nowhere to go, the pressure continued to rise, posing a risk of death. Apparently, if the pressure within the skull becomes greater than the heart's ability to circulate the blood in the brain, then brain death can occur. Fortunately, a skilled brain surgeon (are there unskilled brain surgeons?) put a tube in Clyde's brain to drain the fluid and release the pressure, ultimately saving his life.

Believe it or not, one of the biggest medical complications was bed sores. For some reason, Clyde was not turned, rolled, and moved enough to prevent them. The worst one was at the base of his spine. Once it started, it just got bigger and bigger. Eventually, the salve, light, and medication helped, but the bed sores were a serious problem. For a while, Clyde was put in a bed that blew small round pellets around inside the mattress. Had Clyde been aware of what was happening, he would have had the sensation of floating in air.

In flight training, instructors talk about losing and regaining your orientation. In darkness, it is easy to become disoriented. Sometimes, when it is very dark and the sky is overcast, a pilot can become disoriented and lose ground reference. This means that the pilot might confuse the ground for the sky because the balance centers in the inner ear can become confused as well. Because of an airplane's rapid turn, it can give the pilot a sense of a normal flight path when, in fact, the airplane might be in a steep dive. Of course, the instrument panel can provide valuable information about climbing, turning, and speed. Tragically, some pilots panic, do not believe their instruments, and a disaster is the result. As Clyde gradually came out of his coma, he too was disoriented, not just to his environment but to time, person, and situation as well. Unfortunately, there was no instrument panel to guide him through the mental cloud.

When Clyde's head hit the Cessna's instrument panel, the impact damaged his brain, resulting in memory problems, disorientation, and higher level language deficits. Combined, these problems caused Clyde to act in strange ways. The disorientation experienced by a pilot in darkness is similar to that experienced by a head-trauma patient. For the pilot, disorientation occurs when the demands of the environment exceed his or her knowledge and experience. For Clyde, the mental disorientation he experienced was also because of the interplay between the environment and his cognitive status. The environmental demands exceeded his abilities because of the memory problems, disorientation, and higher level language deficits.

Late one afternoon, Nicole, the air traffic controller at Spring Valley, stopped by the hospital to visit Clyde, her friend of twenty years. He had been moved from the intensive care unit to intermediate care, a step-down unit. Although he was no longer unconscious, his words and actions were bizarre. It was apparent that Clyde did not know where he was or what had happened to him.

Clyde was sitting in a large chair with a table attached to it. To prevent him from escaping or falling over, he was tied to it in an upright position with a sheet. His room was small and the walls were plastered with large-print calendars, pictures of family members, and a blackboard with his daily schedule written in yellow chalk. As Nicole entered the room, the unmistakable odor of a sweaty male was almost overwhelming. But what was indeed overwhelming was what Clyde did next.

When Nicole saw Clyde, she immediately felt a wave of sorrow flood over her. She walked across the room to give him a friendly, supportive hug, and he did something normal Clyde would never do. He grasped her breast and said, in slurred speech that made it seem all the more vulgar, the most offensive thing Nicole had ever heard. Startled, Nicole stepped back and tried to comprehend how Clyde could have been transformed into the monster in the chair. Again, he uttered the offensive statement with a wild-man, profane look on his face. Shocked, Nicole left the room, almost in tears. What had just happened was too much for her to handle. She needed to get away from it all. A nurse saw the startled look on her face and suggested they go to the lounge for a cup of coffee. Nicole consented, hopeful that the nurse could explain what had happened to her friend of twenty years.

The kind nurse explained that Clyde was not responsible for his behavior because he had impaired executive functioning. The brain injury he suffered removed regulatory functions from his personality. With no sense of what was appropriate or inappropriate, Clyde's normal and natural urges had a free reign to control his actions. Clyde's normal sexual urges and needs were not regulated, and his actions simply were a result of this change in his personality. Nicole began to understand that Clyde's behaviors would gradually become more appropriate as he improved, and there was a good likelihood that he would once again be the gentle, polite person she befriended twenty years ago. Sadly, it was unlikely that Clyde would return to complete normalcy. People who suffer serious brain injuries rarely make complete recoveries. But, Nicole learned that Clyde would likely recover many of his thought processes and physical abilities. After the meeting with the nurse, Nicole was optimistic about Clyde's potential. More important, she understood that much of what he was going through was a temporary, and necessary, part of the recovery from a closed-head injury.

Just as the kind nurse predicted, over the next few months Clyde improved considerably. His broken legs healed and some movement returned to his arm. Clyde's memory was still defective, especially for new information, but he was able to manage day-to-day activities. He gradually remembered faces and people from his life before the crash of the Cessna. Ultimately, he was able to live, relatively independently, in a group home not far from the airport where, so many months ago, he began his descent into darkness.

"Murder Challenged"

You see us in airports, malls, movie theaters, and on sidewalks. You hear us talk in restaurants, schools, and churches. But you don't really see us. You don't really hear us. We're like a flutter on the outskirts of your senses. You've been taught not to stare, not to be nosy. When you're forced to acknowledge us, you become nervous, awkward. You speak slowly and loudly. You get very sincere looks on your faces. We're alien to you, and you don't know how to act. You don't know what to say or how to say it.

Oh, I'm not saying you are mean or rude. For the most part, you're not. You just feel uncomfortable around us. Hell, that's understandable. We often feel uncomfortable around you. A long time ago, I began to understand why this happens. I think it is because we're not just different, we're defective. And we're defective in so many different ways. It is frightening to know that our defects easily could have happened, or might still happen, to you. This can be scary and being scared is the worst type of discomfort.

We, the physically and mentally disabled, live in a different world from yours. Ours is a world of shadows, where real participation in your world has been prohibited by God, abnormal genes, birth defects, brain injuries, and spastic muscles. We live on the outskirts of reality town, and we rarely visit Main Street.

Chapter 1

My name is Ben. I'm one of those aliens to your world. I have been one since birth, and I was a big disappointment to my parents. According to the doctors, I was "stressed" during the birth process. Precious molecules of oxygen didn't get to some parts of my brain. The result is me and a disorder known as cerebral palsy. You probably know me as "spaz," "retard," "gimp," or "crip." Those were labels given to me by my brother and hordes of playground bullies. I'm defective because the muscles of my legs, arms, and speech are always tightly pulling against themselves. I spend a lot of time working against myself.

Oh, I'm not mentally deficient. In fact, I have a tested I.Q. that is higher than most or, as they say in statistics, one standard deviation above the norm. My intelligence surprises most people. They just can't accept the fact that I'm not mentally retarded. I suppose it is because I don't appear intelligent. Spastic muscles make my movements slow and awkward. Seeing me shuffle down a concrete sidewalk makes people think that my defects include concrete thinking.

It's my speech that throws most listeners for a loop. Because of those spastic muscles, my talking is labored and distorted, and it really does sound retarded. After hearing me for the first time, almost all listeners respond with slowly spoken, one-word-at-a-time, replies. You know what I'm talking about, the kind of speech reserved for three-year-olds. It's kind of ironic that I'm usually superior in intelligence and education to those talking down to me. Over the years, I've purposefully learned a super vocabulary. I like to see their facial expressions when I say something like, "I'm perplexed with the graphic illustrations of the location of some of the mall's stores.", or "Do you know the shortest distance to the electronics establishment?" It's fun to see the conflicts on the listeners' faces. I can almost hear what they're thinking. "How can this be?" "A retard using complex words?" "Is this candid camera?"

People really get conflicted when, on the first day of class, I walk into the large auditorium classroom and take my place at the podium. I'm sure some of the students think that some retard got confused, accidentally wandered into a university classroom, and some kindly aide will soon remove the creature.

I have had a lot of speech therapy to help me sound more "normal." Quite frankly, I'm sick of all the therapies. As I told Janet, my girlfriend, I've had enough therapy to make a hog puke. Why can't people just accept my "spastic dysarthria," as the medical types call it, as a different dialect or accent? I've heard people from New Orleans and Liverpool, and my accent really isn't much more unusual. Oh well, I'm not a linguist or a social worker. Things are just the way they are, and I'll never be able to change them.

Janet is a very unusual woman. We've been together for almost five years, and I must say, she is something special, and I don't mean "special" in the way people refer to me. To this day, I can't understand why she was ever attracted to me. Each day of my life, I wonder why she stays with me. We've lived together for three years in this small, one bedroom house, not far from her office where she labors with other defectives. She was recently promoted to some type of vocational coordinator and spends a lot of time finding "sheltered" work for the disabled. Janet is good at what she does, and she seems to enjoy it.

Janet isn't one of us. In fact, her body and mind are remarkably flawless. She turned thirty last month, which I noted is fairly old for a woman (this comment was met by her displaying her middle finger in my direction). To undo that unsuccessful attempt at humor, I commented that she has the "aging gracefully" gene. Her jet black hair is void of even one strand of gray, and her skin is as white and smooth as the day she was born. She has long, slender legs and trophy breasts, which appear impervious to gravity. Although she complains of being too fat, she is not overweight. Oh, I'm sure that in the world of skinny super models, where lunch is glass of water and a Saltine (no wonder they always have sour looks on their faces), she would be considered overweight, but in the real world, she is just fine. I appreciate her for what she is. She was blessed with normal limbs and muscles, and a functional brain. As far as I'm concerned she has only one flaw: she appears to have a blind spot. I don't think she sees the defects in me or her clients at work. I wonder if she even perceives us as having flaws. Janet is a very unusual woman, all right.

I'll never forget the first time we met. It was in a course I audited, just for the fun of it, entitled, "The Psychology of Disabilities." It was taught in the evenings by a very normal, middle-aged woman with a degree in psychology. I'll admit, I kind of resented her postulating the psychological effects of disabilities without ever having limped a mile in our shoes. Apparently, we suffer from everything from denial to repressed anger. Some of her ideas were good, but others were pretty lame, at least from my perspective. When some of the more vocal students confronted the professor about her personal lack of knowledge about disabilities, she defended herself by noting that you don't have to have a baby to be a good pediatrician and that giving birth to one doesn't make you an obstetrician. True enough. However, her defense was not good enough for the rest of the disabled in the class, and there were a lot of them. There were quite a few comments about why the university couldn't find a disabled psychologist to teach the class, what with this being the era of affirmative action and all. The good professor managed to fend off the remainder of the attacks and regain control of the class, until she broached the subject of what to call us. That's when the good professor again lost control of her class.

It might not seem a big deal to you, but to the disabled, what we are labeled is important. I suppose a label is big deal to a lot of people, disabled or not. After all, would a doctor want to be called a nurse or a bricklayer called a carpenter? Nowadays, there are a lot of words that set off politically correct debates: Black, Hispanic, Oriental, Right-wing, Gay. Are the meanings of the words "colored people" substantially different from "people of color?" Reasonable or not, these words cause reactions in people. Among the disabled, the semantic reactions occur over words like "disabled," "handicapped," "special," "alternately abled," and "challenged." They set off strong emotions, and sometimes I think countries have gone to war for less. Personally, I don't understand all the hubbub. People should be able to call themselves anything they want as long as it accurately defines them. I prefer to call myself "defective." I am, you know, and no word in English, or any other language, can hide or even minimize that fact. Unfortunately, I don't see many other disabled people rush to use my word. And when I offered it to the class, that is when Janet and I began.

I was brutally attacked by almost the entire class, including the professor. "How could I be so insensitive?" "Why not just call us scum?" "It only focuses on the negative!" Surprised at the heated response from the students, I sat down to lick my wounds when a voice from a wheelchair said, "Shame on you," clearly the work of a speech synthesizer. One student suggested that I be expelled from the class, and there was a hum of general agreement. Geese, what was their problem? Had I not been disabled, I think they would have clubbed me with canes and pinned me to the wall with their wheelchairs.

So, I sat there while the anger saturated the room. My face was flushed and I felt rather embarrassed. Then Janet spoke. She proceeded to give an eloquent speech in defense of me. Her point was that, although she didn't like using the word "defective" to describe people, I had a right to call myself anything I wanted. And who were they to castigate me and my vocabulary? She concluded her Patrick Henry defense of me with the idea that in their politically correct frenzy, they forgot that I have freedom of speech, regardless of how uncomfortable it made them feel. Their uncomfortable feelings were not a sufficient reason to trash the Bill of Rights, to deprive me of my God-given right of expression. Who said college should always be comfortable? Then she sat down, and the professor finally gained control of the classroom.

After class, I made a quick exit. Behind me, I could see hordes of angry, alternately-abled fascists swarming toward me. I was more than a little frightened. I knew they wanted to finish the business started earlier in the class. All I wanted was to escape to my small apartment, swill a beer or two, and try to forget the nightmare that was this class. Thank God, easy egress for the handicapped is not a reality, despite the Americans with Disabilities Act. I managed to outrun the angry hordes. I saw them moving slowly behind me, torches and pitch forks held high, while speech synthesizers droned: "Kill him, Hang him." Well, maybe it wasn't exactly like that, but it was quite a sight nonetheless.

It was a short walk to my apartment, and it was a beautiful autumn evening. Looking behind me, I could see that the mob of politically correct McCarthy's had lost my trail and that I might have time for a fancy coffee. I ducked into a fashionable coffee shop for a decaffeinated latte. As usual, the line was long. There is no such thing as a quick cup of espresso. I patiently stood there waiting my turn, when I heard someone say to me, "I see you got out alive." I turned and there was Janet, and I was forever smitten. I said something to the effect that the class's response to me was "much ado about nothing," and she agreed. I pushed Shakespeare a bit further with a comment about a rose (or stinkweed) by any other name. I thanked her for coming to my defense, even though I was perfectly capable of it, had I not been so startled by their anger. She graciously accepted my qualified thanks, and we sat together at one of those miniature tables seen in coffee shops around the world. For the next couple of hours we talked, discussed, argued, and laughed. I learned about her and she about me. They were two of the most satisfying hours of my life. As we left the coffee shop, I had her telephone number firmly tucked away in my wallet.

About two days later, I mustered the courage to call Janet. I was going to wait longer, say three or four days, but I was too caught up in the excitement of possibilities. So, I ran the risk of appearing too eager, rang her up, as they say in England, and was both surprised and delighted when she accepted my proposition of a movie and dinner. Actually, after the phone call, I felt a little disappointed. Janet so readily accepted my invitation, so eagerly agreed to go out with me, that I began to wonder what was wrong with her. What major personality flaw did she have? What kind of woman would be so eager to go out with a defective like me? I'm painfully aware that I'm not the most attractive man in the world, what with my spastic muscles and all. And even if my muscles would relax, I'm still not blessed with the features most women swoon over.

And then there is my personality. I never bought into the idea that just because my passage through my mother's birth canal was a major headache, I should forever be humble, quiet and reserved in thought and actions. I was never the kind to sit quietly on the outskirts and to know my place in normal society. Quite frankly, I adopted my attitude at an early age: "Screw the huddled masses and their superior, self-righteous beliefs about me and my kind." I simply believe that even with my defects I'm as good or better than most. I also don't take life and disabilities so seriously. I usually see the humorous side of most things and that includes the world of the handicapped. I have been called a "spastic with an attitude." So, given my obvious physical flaws and not so obvious personality ones, I was, at first, disappointed at Janet for agreeing to go out with someone like me. I would have to examine her very closely for fatal feminine flaws.

Luckily, I am able to drive my specially equipped van. It's quite a machine. I have easy access to the steering apparatus and other essential control systems, including my state-of-the-art stereo system. The van didn't need major modifications. It cost a pretty penny, but it is well worth it. I purposefully chose the brightest red paint, fanciest wheels, and a 440 cubic inch powerhouse motor, because I wanted it to be more of a rod than a dark, dreary machine you see in handicapped parking spaces. Last year, I had dual glass-packed mufflers put on. I just love to hear the engine start. I swear it growls, like an angry lion with a bad case of hemorrhoids. I know, I'm a little long in the tooth to be excited about mufflers and engines, but I suppose if I can have arrested development, it can include this teenage fancy for big engines and loud mufflers.

Janet was impressed with the rod all right. I think she was a little surprised, too. Where did I get the money for tuck and roll leather seats, oversized tires, and all of the other options and accessories? She knew I was a professor on campus, and I'm also certain she knew that professors, especially third-year assistant ones like me, didn't make big bucks.

I don't tell people that I am a published novelist, a writer of mysteries. I even write them under a pseudonym. When I say I'm published, I mean I have had two books actually hit the bookstores. My first book, *Murder in Montana*, didn't quite shake the world of publishing with its sales. Sixteen hundred books were sold and most of them to libraries. Didn't quite hit the *New York Times* bestsellers list with my first try. But my second book, *A Death in Denver*, surprised me and my publisher, who I think only published my books because I'm disabled, a kind of politically correct novelty act that can be boasted about in corporate meetings. But, surprise, surprise, as Gomer Pyle would say, I sold over a hundred thousand copies of my second book. It's now in its third printing, and twice a year, I get rewarded handsomely for it. I get 10% of the net sales, minus returns, for the first 10,000 copies, and 12% for any books sold beyond that. So I get a couple bucks for each book, and when you sell thousands of them, it adds up. My van was the first purchase I made with the royalty checks.

As planned, Janet and I had our first real date. The movie was yet another coming-of-age, sophomore romp, where teenage boys desperately and clumsily seek their first sexual experience. Although the plot was predictable and the bathroom humor only marginally laughable, we had a wonderful time. Janet alternately laughed and was disgusted at the appropriate times. We ordered the same meal at dinner, which was the required first-date fare of a northern Italian plate of fishy pasta with a pretentious name and too much garlic. Although our first date was less than unique, we enjoyed ourselves with easy conversation and comfortable interaction. Never did I detect the slightest aversion to my physical and speech defects and, in fact, Janet initiated the always awkward good-night kiss. Sadly, there was no invitation to late-night-coffee-sex in her apartment, but the kiss alone sustained me. Driving home, I knew I had met the woman of my dreams, one I would pursue until I was thoroughly rejected.

During the fall semester, we shared more sophomore movies, pasta plates, and awkward kisses. I grew to love everything about her. I was hopelessly mesmerized by this wonderful, strange creature who accepted me for me. We met for coffee, walked along the Oak River, and talked and talked on the telephone and via e-mail. Once, while standing in line at "our" coffee shop, we both overheard a seven-year-old girl ask her mother why I walked and talked so funny. Of course, I have heard questions and comments like these almost daily since I was old enough to understand them. I have learned to ignore most of them, and the hurtful ones, I have rationalized. I was delighted when Janet appeared either to immediately forget the comment or to ignore it altogether. She appeared to have the indifference, the thick-skinned attitude, that was going to be necessary if she were to spend more time with me. I knew that as long as we were together, there would be many more of them. To respond to them is simply a waste of time and energy. Nothing will ever stop them, so all I can do is control my reactions, and I'm getting very good at it. I am almost impervious to them.

People don't like talking about sex and the disabled. Hell, most people won't even allow themselves to think about it, although our society is preoccupied with sex. It permeates our movies, books, and television shows. Old people remember it, and the young ones can't talk about anything else. Our billboards, magazine ads, and television snippets use it to sell us everything from tires to toilet paper. But you never see sex and the disabled together. Society would rather think of us as asexual creatures. Oh, I understand it. If our physical bodies distress the good senses of the normal world, then imagining us in the act of sex must be a mental toothache. On a deeper level, there is the primal fear that reproduction among or with the disabled would propagate only the worst of the gene pool. I think most people believe that only a sick normal person would even consider sex with a defective.

Janet is one sick person. Not only did she consider sex with me, she appeared to thoroughly enjoy every aspect of it. She liked it, and she liked it with her eyes wide open and with the lights on. The first time I was understandably self-conscious, but not Janet. She was initiator, facilitator, and in many ways, a competitor. She was also very goal-oriented, which became pleasurably apparent when she whispered, "I'm not done with you."

Chapter 2

Lazlow Price carefully prepared the potion in his dimly lit room on Milton Avenue. He could hear the cars whirl past his window, with hurried drivers blasting horns, screeching tires, and gunning engines. Morning rush hour was the loudest, and he welcomed the noise. The noise was good, even when it kept him awake at night. It really didn't matter, the noise that is, because it had been years since Lazlow had slept an entire night. The nightmares always came and brought a quick end to his rest. Images of disgusting creatures filled his nighttime reprieve. God-awful crips, retards, and droolers slowly approached him in nightmare after nightmare, trying to sap his strength. They would take and take until there was nothing left, and if he didn't startle to awaken, sweating and fearful, they would take it all, his limbs, his mind, and ultimately his life.

Lazlow really didn't hate them. He really didn't hate mosquitoes, rats, or nighttime barking dogs either. A well-timed slap, mousetrap, or .22 caliber bullet usually eliminated the problem. They were just problems with easy solutions, and it was his duty, even his calling in life, to eliminate them. It was also his pleasure. As he used an eyedropper to place the last of the poison in the vile, he knew he was doing God's work, and that thought fortified and energized him. Tomorrow, he would begin the crusade. Tomorrow, Lazlow Price would begin the extermination of human vermin. He would protect normal, God-fearing people, the gene pool, and a society that did not know how to make the hard decisions. Tomorrow, he would kill, exterminate really, a life that had no right to live, a life better off dead. As the traffic noise gradually died down, the short, balding, overweight chemistry major with thick, Coke-bottle glasses, continued to concoct a poison that could not easily be detected in a routine autopsy and that was virtually tasteless. His professors and the Net had taught him well.

Lazlow's part-time day job was completely free from responsibility. He simply poured liquids into bowls, cups, and glasses, and plopped meats and fixings onto plates. Five or six hours a day, with two breaks and one lunch hour, he performed this function for hundreds of loud, demanding, hurried students. His coworkers performed the same tasks and rarely spoke to him; their only commonality was the black, spider web hair nets. The job had been tolerable until the powers that be had hired one of these disgraces to humanity to perform the identical tasks. She was one of them, and Lazlow knew she must be exterminated.

Chapter 3

It is one of the largest universities in the country. It boasts one of the most populous dormitory complexes and the largest college bus system. There are miles and miles of paved bicycle roads with passing lanes and traffic signs. The university proudly supports three medical schools (human, osteopathic, and veterinary) and a world-famous law school. With strong agricultural roots, it invents new fertilizers, pesticides and herbicides, and genetically engineered fruits and vegetables. You can even buy "chocolate cheese," obtained somehow from contented campus cows, from a small shop next to the International Center. The International Center is the hub of the campus, located next to the official campus bookstore and housing several specialty stores, dining rooms, coffee shops, and cafes. From it, you can see the library complex towering over the campus and housing more volumes than any other college in the Midwest. You can hear Bell Tower announce the hour and half hour throughout the university and surrounding townships. The campus is lush with trees, grass, bushes, and colorful flowers. The university is a city unto itself. It has its own fire and police departments, preschools, hospitals, and clinics. It dominates the small town that physically surrounds it. Campus and town borders are blurred and, economically, the university is a parasite, drawing apartments, food and beer from the small, grateful community.

During the fall semester, acres of oak and maple trees brightly color the campus. Fifty thousand students swarm the grounds and buildings, soaking up the rich education offered. It is a liberal campus, tolerant of everything but intolerance and, sometimes, freedom of expression. It also serves as a magnet for those students and nonstudents on the fringe of mental stability. On this campus and ones like it, dangerous mental illnesses can be disguised as just another unique way of looking at the world.

The Oak River flows slowly through the southern part of the campus. You can rent canoes and watch ducks, muskrats, beavers, and turtles do what they have done since the land-grant college was legislated into existence. The river winds through the huge groves of trees to a small, unincorporated township where Ma and Pa sell world-class, homemade ice cream. Canoeing upstream is as easy as downstream because the Oak River takes its time and forces reflection and relaxation on all who venture on it.

Clarene and Donna liked to watch the canoes being launched and captured at the dock. This green spot, next to a huge flowering rose bush, was a favorite lunch hour place for the two day-workers to leisurely eat their homemade sandwiches. On the grassy knoll, high above the dock, they would sit, eat, and take in the beauty the campus had to offer. There was always a comical landing where a canoe would slam into the dock or other canoes, and clumsy, unsure passengers would scramble to the safety of wooden planks. Twice, they had witnessed passengers slip or fall into the muddy river, waist deep in embarrassment. Clarene and Donna would never laugh at the wet unfortunates, they were not rude, but they would silently enjoy the lunch hour slapstick nonetheless. Sometimes, back at the apartment, the roommates would recount the events on the Oak River and chuckle, but never meanly. They simply enjoyed seeing normal people, out of their element, stumble, slip, and slide when trying to negotiate water and land obstacles. Clarene was always out of her element. Leg braces and cumbersome, primitive crutches helped, but awkwardness was always a part of her life.

Clarene was older than Donna by three years. At 22, she had long ago accepted her physical self. That her spine was deformed at birth was simply a fact of her life. She no longer dreamed of a cure. She was what she was and that was it. Acceptance had not come easily, but it had come. Clarene was perfectly at ease with herself. Sometimes she even wondered, if offered a miracle cure, would she take it? She liked herself. Sometimes, when she knew no one would see, she would stare at herself in the full-length mirror in the hall. She was blessed with so many things beautiful. Her long, blond, slightly curly hair ornamented her pleasant facial features and velveteen skin. She wore little makeup because there was little to make up. She had a typical hourglass frame, at least to her hips. She seldom allowed herself to look below her thin waist at the deformed lower back and legs. Oh, she didn't deny their existence, she simply focused on the many positive aspects of her youthful body. Clarene was an optimist.

Donna was a sweet girl. Actually, at nineteen, she was more woman than girl. Down syndrome had given her the physical characteristics once called "Mongoloid." Her round face and slightly slanted eyes made her resemble Chinese Mao more than Nordic Sven, but the oriental reference had long ago slipped from most people's vocabulary. Down syndrome had restricted Donna to the mental age of a ten-year-old. She did everything like a ten-year-old: read, write, speak and think. Oh, she was a delightful ten-year-old, but a ten-year-old nonetheless. The only unsettling thing about Donna was that she had the body of a young woman. A ten-year-old managing a woman's body.

Janet had negotiated intensely with the reluctant food service company to employ Clarene and Donna. Actually, they had hired Clarene on the spot but needed coaxing, planning, and reassurance to hire Donna. Spraying hot water over dirty cups, plates, and pots was an ideal job for Clarene. She could sit, spray, and then push the tray through the state-of-the-art dishwashing machine. Confident legs were not necessary to succeed at this job in the food service industry. But finding a job for Donna was more difficult. Janet had almost given up on gainful employment for the ten/nineteen-year-old when she saw how the plastic spoons, knives, and forks had been sorted and carefully wrapped in paper napkins. Instantly, she knew that this was a job easily performed by the ten-year-old in the young woman's body. The food service manager had finally agreed, and later, other similar jobs were added, including stacking the clean cups, plates, and pots that were rinsed by Clarene. To everyone surprise but Janet's, both women were now in their second year of minimum-wage employment. The satisfied food service manager had even remarked that she would be willing to hire more job-hopefuls from the shelter.

"He's kinda scary," confided Clarene, nodding in the direction of the balding, overweight coworker pouring apple, orange, and grapefruit juices into small glasses. Donna glanced in his direction and smiled in agreement. Of course, for Donna, many men were scary, not so much because of their words and actions but because of the feelings they stirred in her. Very unusual and disquieting feelings. Sometimes, when men stood close to her, she almost tingled with a strange anticipation of something exciting and unknown. She had never told Clarene that the man called "Laz" by the rest of the staff had made her tingle more than most men. The 19-year-old Donna was attracted to the man, and the ten-year-old Donna didn't understand why or where it would lead.

Several times Donna had approached Laz in an awkward, innocent attempt to spark a deeper relationship, and every time, he had rebuffed her. The rebuffs took many forms, not making eye-contact, walking away midsentence, feigning work demands. His seething contempt for her and her kind was not readily apparent to the other workers or to Donna, for that matter. Today, however, Laz was uncharacteristically gracious and friendly.

During the morning break, both sat together in the employee lounge, apparently enjoying small talk. When Donna went to the restroom, no one saw Laz quickly open her plastic water container, empty the vile of poison in it, tighten the cap, and carefully replace it in her small backpack, sitting next to her brown bag lunch with a ham and cheese sandwich, chips, and an apple.

The small family who lived in a rundown married housing unit had enjoyed the noontime sojourn down Oak River. Robert, a graduate student soon to complete his oral defense of a dissertation exploring a filter's ability to remove e-coli bacteria from water, helped his young, pregnant wife, and two-year-old son disembark from the narrow, wobbly canoe. As the three-soon-to-be-four family finally stood secure on the dock, they heard the screams from atop the grassy knoll. Immediately, Robert ran to the aid of the distressed woman knowing that he might be able to help, given his training as an EMT. It had paid most of his undergraduate expenses, thus keeping his student loans to a minimum. Reaching the top of the knoll, it was soon apparent that the teenager lying on the grass was in full respiratory arrest. Robert quickly began CPR, which proved to be too little, too late. By the time the ambulance arrived, Donna was dead, even though the CPR continued during the ride to the hospital. That sunny midday, sweet Donna's body was sent to the morgue, and the awful business of informing relatives and friends of a young woman's premature demise was begun. Janet was the first at the shelter to be given the shocking news.

Chapter 4

Every day that Steven Thompson patrolled the campus, he was aware of the lack of respect, the outright disregard the students had for the campus police. The students, and most of the faculty and staff too, regarded the campus police as cop "wannabes." They simply did not accept the campus police as "real" cops, a perception that was a thorn in the side of most members of the force. That Steven, and the rest of the campus police department, had the same qualifications as most cops and had completed rigorous training and education programs didn't seem to be general information on this campus, with an enrollment larger than many cities. And when it came to the real power of the campus police, they carried, and used if necessary, the same pistols and riot control arsenals cops in New York or Los Angeles were issued. Most importantly, the campus police had the same powers to stop, detain, and arrest suspects. This campus police department even had a one man detective division, and Steven was it.

Steven was tall, almost too tall for the force. Fortunately, he had missed the maximum height limit by an inch. As the only plainclothes policeman, he was not required to wear a uniform. However, Steven took pride in his appearance, always wearing a tie and sport coat and ever conscious about the shine on his shoes. His moustache was the only thing about his appearance that was not standard police issue, and it was beginning to show signs of gray. At forty-seven, Steven had been in law enforcement for half of his life. The first years were spent as a military policeman and then twelve years with the police department in Laramie, Wyoming. He had been with the campus police more than nine years and was looking forward to completing his career as a campus detective.

Steven had stuttered most of his adult life. In fact, he had stuttered since the third grade. He didn't remember the exact date the stuttering began or what event caused it, he simply remembered it beginning when he was about eight. The stuttering problem wasn't a severe one, it was barely noticeable most of the time. There were occasions when speech was impossible, but they happened infrequently, and then only when he felt a lot of stress. Most of the time, Steven just repeated the first sounds of words too many times and occasionally stretched out a word here and there. During severe bouts with the speech disorder, Steven would feel his vocal cords close off and stop the air and sounds coming from his mouth. Eventually, the words would come but only after long, embarrassing, and anxious moments.

The 911 call from the Oak River boat dock came in about 12:30 p.m. The student-wage dispatcher had sent the ambulance winding through the crowded campus streets, and he had also notified Steven and the closest cruiser. Steven had just completed the paperwork on two students caught with a marijuana bong in their dorm room. The lab analysis had shown enough residual pot to suspend them from school and to require them to attend a drug information program. He knew the Dean of Students wouldn't expel them, and that was fine. After all, it was just pot and just carelessness that had resulted in the arrest. A simple slap on the hands was all that was necessary, not that it would do any good in preventing drug abuse by thousands of students. It would simply require them to be more careful about getting caught.

As the senior policeman on campus, Steven got to use the new white, unmarked sedan that was recently purchased by the reluctant administration. It had been hard to convince the administration, and the faculty law enforcement committee, that the department needed the unmarked car. But after three years of pleading, Steven had finally prevailed. When he arrived at the grassy knoll, the ambulance was loading the young woman and futile CPR was being given in earnest. Later, he learned from the intake nurse in the emergency room that the teenager was DOA. He took statements from two students, a married couple who lived on campus and who had been at the dock when the death had occurred. He also interviewed the young woman's roommate, who had been picnicking with her. She was in her early twenties and had been understandably upset. Steven was happy to give the handicapped woman a ride to the hospital and then to her apartment complex.

The dead woman was one of those disabled people you sometimes see on campus. Most were students, but some simply worked at menial tasks in dorms or dinning rooms. He had noted that she had Down syndrome and had remembered from some distant conversation that many of the people with this chromosome disorder did not live long lives. Her roommate, Clarene, had informed him that early death was no longer a necessary fate for Down syndrome sufferers. Medical advances had prevailed, and many now lived long lives. However, the medical examiner determined the cause of death to be a simple heart attack, probably as a result of a preexisting valve irregularity. For Steven, this sad event was opened and closed with little fanfare. People die, and the handicapped are not immune from dying young, despite medical advances.

Chapter 5

Janet couldn't believe the news of Donna's death. That such an innocent, pleasant young woman could die so young, so unexpectedly, was a shock to every staff member at the center, especially Janet. But what was even more devastating to Janet was the difficult task of breaking the news to the clients, especially the ones with lower intelligence. For some, the concept of mortality was beyond their reach; for others, the bad news would only be partially understood. Of course, because Janet was the favorite of the clients, the role of bearer of the bad new was her responsibility, one she dreaded.

For the people who had only a passing familiarity with Donna, the news was given in small groups. The others, the ones that had been her friends, Janet met with them individually. By evening, all of the clients in the shelter knew of Donna's premature demise. That night, Janet went home exhausted to the comfort of Ben and bed. He prepared the late dinner, then held and quietly listened to her into the early morning. They made love and slept the light sleep of mourners, dreading the morning sun and another day of grief.

Two months later, Lazlow Price worked late into the night, again preparing the death potion. Pleased that his first extermination had been a success, he planned the next act of social cleansing. He knew his job as a food server provided him with unlimited opportunities to dispense death. Since discovering a method of time-release for the poison, another marvelous fact obtained from the Net, Lazlow knew the chances of the police tracing the deaths back to him was remote. Time-released liquids, one of the newest pharmacological miracles, were being used in cough syrups and other liquid medicines, and it was relatively easy for Lazlow to delay the fatal effects of his poison by over an hour.

Lazlow had seen his next victim only a few times. Probably because he had new courses in buildings next to the International Center, the soon-to-be-dead student in a wheelchair had started coming to the cafe for his usual cup of coffee and bagel. Each time Lazlow saw him in line and served him coffee, he could barely hide his repulsion. Thoroughly disgusted, Lazlow would give him a banana nut bagel and coffee. Today, however, the coffee was more than a beverage. It was a death drug that in an hour or so, would cleanse the world of yet another despicable creature.

Chapter 6

Although I teach courses in literature, I can't actually say I'm a professor. I teach only one course at a time, and I'm not on that road to happiness known as a tenure track. Quite frankly, I don't care about tenure or promotion that much. Part time work is just fine with me, and given my latest book royalties, I'm happy just teaching one course a term. I get to teach a subject I enjoy and get to meet interesting students.

I have a policeman in one of my courses. Actually, he's only a campus cop, but he seems quite competent nonetheless. Over the year, we've become friends. We both look forward to a cup of coffee after class at the International Center, where we discuss things related to major British writers. To complete his liberal studies' requirements, he is taking my course, and last semester, he took my twentieth-century writers course. He's an unusual student, not only because he's older but because his law enforcement experience makes for very interesting discussions.

I wasn't surprised when he told me of the death of the Mongoloid girl. A death on a university campus usually involves a lot of people, and most students and faculty are touched by the rumor mill. When he told me of meeting Janet, and I informed him of our "live-in" status, we made the "small world" comments necessitated by such a coincidence. The world of coincidence got smaller when he told me of the death of another disabled person.

Apparently, a wheelchair-bound man had also died of a heart attack or something. Steven told me about the events surrounding his death. The thirty-year-old had been in a motorcycle accident when he was in his teens. His spine had been broken, severing the all-important cord that links the brain to the body. He was paralyzed from the waist down and used a state-of-the-art motorized wheelchair to get from place to place. Last year, he had enrolled at the University and was seeking a degree in History and Political Science, with the goal of taking the Law School Admissions Test and becoming a lawyer. He was going to a morning class on south campus when his wheelchair plowed into several students. He was hunched over, dead at the controls.

That evening, I told Janet of the demise of yet another disabled person. Although he was not a client at the shelter, she had also heard of his death. We both commented that two deaths occurring in such a short time was unusual.

Chapter 7

Lazlow thought how easy it was to kill them. He doubted the authorities ever thought their deaths were from anything other than natural causes, natural causes for creatures that were unfit to live in the first place. It was so easy. So clean. So effective. But, the ease of his extermination plan was beginning to bother him too. There was no lesson for society to learn and, worst of all, no gratitude for a job well done. Early one evening, while the rush-hour traffic moaned outside his apartment, Lazlow decided to be more bold, more obvious, and more lethal. He decided to make public his extermination goals. He would not only exterminate an undesirable, he would make a social statement. And to make it public, he would call the student newspaper and announce his intent.

Lazlow both dreaded and was intrigued by the "Major British Writers" liberal studies course he was required to take. He was intrigued by the idea of killing the well-liked professor. As he watched the professor shuffle to the podium, Lazlow silently planned his next extermination. It was one that would undoubtedly bring him national attention and the praise and recognition he deserved. Death would be swift and true, and the campus would buzz with the event within minutes of the deed. Lazlow felt excitement and pride at the act he would perform. He listened to the raspy voice he would silence as the disgusting professor waxed on and on about Chaucer and the writer's perspectives on life and morality, and the filth of the *Canterbury Tales*. After work, on the walk back to his noisy apartment, Lazlow stopped at a public phone and called the student newspaper. As expected, because it was after hours, he spoke to an answering machine. He calmly read the short, prepared statement from a crumpled sheet of paper he had tucked away in his pocket:

> I am the exterminator of defectives. The world is purer by the death of two life forms. The next defective to be exterminated sings the praises of a British pornographer. His voice will be silenced. Praise be to the Lord.

Lazlow hung up the phone and continued the walk to his apartment in the cool fall air.

The *State News* is run by students, mostly journalism majors. Of course, there is the faculty advisor, Professor Jennifer Johnson, who serves more as a censor than advisor. When Professor Johnson heard the recording of the exterminator's threat, she knew it shouldn't be taken lightly. The *State News* had run stories about the deaths of both disabled people, and she remembered them clearly. Both articles stated that the deaths were the results of natural causes. Now, the advisor was not certain. After the excited student who had brought her the answering machine tape had left, she called the campus police.

After meeting with Professor Johnson, Steven Thompson called the Federal Bureau of Investigation and spoke to an impatient receptionist who had little tolerance for his stutter. Treating him as if he were retarded, she finally connected him to the appropriate special agent for the region. Steve wondered how special an agent was if every agent in the Bureau was called "special." By the next day, the small campus police headquarters was crowded by clean-cut, suit-wearing F.B.I. agents, "fibies" as they were called in Wyoming, trained to deal with homicides and death threats. Within hours of their arrival, a judge had ordered exhumation of Donna's and the pre-law student's bodies. The extensive autopsies conducted by the F.B.I. pathologist found traces of the poison that caused their deaths. On the death certificates, demise from "natural causes" was now changed to "homicide." The murder investigations began in earnest.

Chapter 8

After reading the *State News* article about the death threat, I began to feel uneasy. In the recesses of my mind, I entertained the idea that I might be next on the hitman's list. I was certainly a candidate. I was disabled, on campus, and highly visible. At dinner that evening, Janet also noted that many students consider some of the *Canterbury Tales* sexually explicit, and some might even consider them pornography. Was it a coincidence that in the past week my lectures were about Chaucer?

Initially, Steven downplayed my concerns, but as we talked about motives and opportunities, he, too, began to suspect that I might be next. The following day we met in my office and went over the list of students in my Major British Writers course. I had one section of the course, with a total enrollment of more than 150. Steven methodically scanned the enrollment roster for names of students with any criminal history. Two students were found to have a rap sheet, but both offenses were for driving under the influence. A third student had been arrested for shoplifting in her freshman year. All three students were eliminated as possible suspects. By afternoon, we both had accepted the fact that I was vulnerable and that my fears were real. Steven said I should seriously consider canceling my course and remaining in my apartment or leaving town until the murderer was apprehended. The minute he made the suggestions that I run and hide from harm's way, I knew it would never happen.

I'm simply not the kind of person to run from a threat. Maybe it is because of my disabilities. I have never been able to run from them, either. They're real and ever present. It has been my experience that you either confront and deal with them, or you forever run. And the running is not really from them, it is from yourself, and there is no place to hide. I have found that you must embrace all that is you, the good, the bad, and the ugly. We don't live in a perfect world, and there are few of us who even approach perfection. As Popeye so philosophically noted, "I yam what I yam, and that's all I yam." Well, if there is a crazed killer out there determined to eliminate me, then so be it. I'll do what I can to prevent it. Hell, I do everything I can to keep living, but I won't run and hide. It's not in my constitution. I just won't do it.

Steven and I listened to the tape with the terse threat on it, hoping I might be able to recognize the voice. But with over 150 students, it was futile, mostly because I have never met the majority of my students, let alone had a conversation with them. My class is a standard lecture one, "a sage on stage," as some call it. Occasionally, a student will ask a question or offer a comment, but even that is a rare occurrence. The course is held three times a week, with each lecture lasting fifty minutes. It's not an interactive course; there is very little student participation.

In my first novel, *Murder in Montana*, I had done some research on speech recognition devices. The plot of the novel revolved around a corporate employee who had stolen and sold the formula for a powerful antidote to several lethal gases that were used in the Gulf War. He had then changed his identity and, with the profits from selling the secret of the antidote, moved to West Yellowstone, Montana to enjoy the spoils of his crime. During the research for the book, I discovered that many high-tech companies were using two types of identification systems to allow selective access to secret computer files. A widely used authorization device is a retina scan. Laser light scans a person's retina and because no two are identical, positive identification can be made. Once the domain of science fiction, retina scanning has now become relatively commonplace in high-tech companies and governmental agencies.

The second type of identification is through voice prints. Similar to retinas, no two individuals' voices and speech patterns are identical. Voice prints are more useful than retina scans because most computers, even laptops, have embedded microphones that permit this type of speaker recognition. All a person has to do is speak a series of words, which have been previously analyzed, into the microphone, and the computer then either denies or allows access to documents and data, based on the acoustical analysis. In my novel, access to the antidote formula was permitted using this type of device.

Steven and I were convinced that the murderer was a member of my Major British Writers course. First, he had used the word "defectives." In my courses, I sometimes jokingly refer to myself as a defective when I drop lecture notes or chalk or have to repeat myself due to my speech disorder. I say something like, "Pardon my defective speech," or "It's not easy being a defective." These comments usually bring lighthearted laughter to the classroom and make the students feel more at ease with me and my disabilities. Second, the murderer had made the pornography comment, this occurring during my lectures on Chaucer. Given, all of this is circumstantial evidence at best, but at least it was something. Steven and I agreed that if we could somehow get a voice sample from each student, we could compare them to the answering machine tape. The big problem was how to obtain a speech sample with one or more of the words used on the threatening tape. For accurate analysis, the same word has to be used for comparison purposes.

Steven and I carefully analyzed the transcript of the answering machine tape. How could I get all 150 students to say one or more of the words on the tape? *I am the exterminator of defectives. The world is purer by the death of two life forms. The next defective to be exterminated sings the praises of a British pornographer. His voice will be silenced. Praise be to the Lord.* My first thought was the word "I." It is the most frequently used word in English. But how to get the students to say it? Steven and I sat stooped over the sample for hours until, in frustration, we decided to sleep on it. After all, I had to prepare the midterm examination.

Sometimes in my sleep I solve problems. I understand that this is not necessarily unusual. Many people wake up with a solution to a nagging problem. I have heard that even Einstein solved a major mathematical problem in his sleep. Somehow, during sleep, the mind is free to explore options or to allow solutions to surface. And maybe, because I'm disabled, the freedom of dreaming is more important in problem-solving. That morning at precisely 4:30, it hit me. I woke Janet and told her of the solution, as much to share the revelation as to ensure that I would not go back to sleep and forget it.

As soon as Steven got to his office, I called and told him of my plan. I would get a speech sample from all of the students during the examination. I also resolved to keep my investigation from the F.B.I. I doubted my plan would be constitutional.

When Lazlow Price read the small *State News* article about the death threat, he became furious. It was just a small article, hidden on page nine of the paper. Worst of all, no local television or newspapers picked it up. What infuriated Lazlow more than anything was that they didn't take him seriously. Apparently, to them, he was just another crackpot. Well, he resolved, they'll be taught a lesson and soon.

Chapter 9

The Department of Speech and Hearing Sciences is located on the third floor of Building 6 in the Health Sciences Complex. Steven and I had made an appointment to meet with one of the professors who was knowledgeable about voice prints. Dr. Oscar Sciacca, a senior faculty member and specialist in the acoustics of speech, expressed immediate interest in our situation and said he could compare the voice prints of the 150 students. He would use two research assistants to help with the tedious aspects of preparing the voice samples. As we walked with him to his laboratory, he asked the whys, whats and wherefores about the project. Steven provided him with the detailed information about the death threat and how we intended to get the voice samples. Dr. Sciacca suggested we get the actual telephone and answering machine from the *State News* office because he would need them to do the analysis of the speech samples. Apparently, telephones and tape recorders vary in their frequency responses. He also wanted the tape recorder we would be using to obtain the speech samples from the students.

Examination day is stressful for everyone, students, teaching assistants, and professors alike. Today was no exception, especially since I suspected that one of my students was planning to murder me. Once the students had filed into my classroom, I had my two teaching assistants distribute the computer grading sheets to them. As soon as they settled down, I briefly welcomed them to the class and asked that they fill in the blanks and darken the small dots indicating their name, seat, and social security numbers. While they were busily working their number two pencils, I casually took three photographs of the classroom with my small camera.

After the doors were closed and locked, my teaching assistants began distributing the examination. The students believed there were several forms of this examination and they, upon receiving the exam, needed to tell the teaching assistants which one they had. Prior to distributing the exam, I had written the words "Form Two" at the top of first page of every test. I told the students that because of computer problems, they must tell the teaching assistants their names and which form they received. Because I wanted them to have the full fifty minutes to finish the exam, they would speak their names and form numbers into a small digital tape recorder held about six inches from their lips. The teaching assistant would then have a record of the student's name and form number to ensure proper grading of the exams. I apologized for the computer glitch but assured them that it was necessary if grading was to be accurate. I made up a phony story about the problems the Central Scanning department was having with their new hardware. As the students received their tests, each one spoke his or her name and the same words, "Form Two," into the tape recorder held by the teaching assistants.

No student questioned the change in testing protocol and this didn't surprise me. The students were simply too preoccupied with remembering the information, completing the exam, and getting home for much needed sleep after hours of cramming. The collecting of speech samples was completed without a hitch. Three students had left messages on my voice-mail indicating they could not take the examination at the designated time because of family emergencies or illnesses. Fortunately, all three were female, and we excluded them from the suspect list.

Steven was waiting for me at my office when I returned after the last test had been completed by the slowest student. I thought it was overkill and a little dramatic, but Steven used the siren and flashing portable light of his car to get us to Dr. Sciacca's lab. He and his two assistants were analyzing the speech samples within fifteen minutes of our arrival. Steven would wait at the speech acoustics lab while I took the film to be developed. I knew there was a one-hour photo shop in the International Center. I called Janet from my cell phone as I walked past the libraries. She agreed to meet with me and have a cup of decaffeinated latte at "our" coffee shop in the International Center. We frequently met there after my class. It was sort of a pleasant ritual begun years ago when we first started dating.

Steven offered to help Dr. Sciacca and the lab assistants. They politely refused his help, and he silently wondered if it was because of his stutter. During the past week or so, it had been getting worse, probably a result of the stress he was feeling about the murders and danger Ben was in. He had always admired Ben for his intellect. He was one of the most intelligent people he'd ever met. Now, he also admired him for his courage. Steven saw him differently since he'd refused to stay home or leave the campus until the murderer was caught. Oh, he knew Ben was afraid, but he wasn't about to let some crackpot make him run and hide. He wouldn't buckle. Steven knew Ben saw the murderer much like he viewed his own disabilities. Ben would confront these trials and tribulations much like he did his cerebral palsy—straight ahead. Ben was a courageous man.

A voice print breaks the speech signal into three components: time, frequency, and energy. The computer readout, called a spectrogram, shows small, detailed aspects of these three aspects. Although all words have basic similarities in time, frequency, and energy, there are minor individual variations among different speakers. One way of looking at it is that a person's head is a resonating chamber, much like a musical instrument such as a violin or trombone. The vocal cords serve as a source of vibration and certain aspects of that energy is amplified or dampened by a person's head. And because people's heads, or resonating chambers, are different, their spectrograms are different. Even identical twins have different spectrograms because, though their heads are identical, they have learned to speak differently. For example, one twin might produce the /s/ sound a little longer in duration than the other twin. These differences are in milliseconds. Also, there might be small differences between the length of pauses between sounds, the way voice onset occurs, or how the pitch rises at the end of a vowel in anticipation of another sound. These are a result of individual learning, and no two people share all of them. There are many other little variations that can be detected. Voice print analysis consists of looking at these resonance and speech pattern differences for consistency. In the past, the analysis took days, even weeks, but now they are rapidly and accurately done by computers.

About an hour after the voice analyses began, Dr. Sciacca and his assistants made a positive match. Speech sample eleven, a male by the name of Lazlow Price, had a 95% positive match with the word "Form" and a 97%

accuracy value with the word "Two." Steven immediately logged onto the police department's computer and searched the records for a Mr. Lazlow Price. He found no wants or warrants and no significant rap sheet other than three parking violations. He then searched the administration records and found that the suspect had several student loans and part-time employment at one of the cafes in the International Center. In fact, it was a coffee shop frequented by Ben, who was probably there now waiting for the film to be developed. Ben had a weakness for decaffeinated latte. Suddenly, Steven feared for his friend's life.

As Steven rushed to his car, he tried several times to call Ben on his cell phone. There was no answer. Ben must have forgotten to turn it on. As he sped through the narrow campus streets with siren blasting and light flashing, he had the dispatcher send a cruiser to the coffee shop. He doubted the cruiser would beat him there, but this was one of those situations where time definitely was of the essence.

Janet was already at a table sipping her coffee. Actually, she was sipping the whipped cream generously plopped atop it. I ordered my usual from one of the familiar faces doing the serving and soon was sitting next to my beautiful girlfriend. In the distance, I could hear the "wherrrr" of a siren and assumed another pedestrian had been clipped at an intersection, a frequent and unfortunate occurrence on this busy campus. As I reached for my first sip of coffee, my spastic muscles caused an overshooting of movement, and I spilled some of the hot beverage on my lap, not exactly an unusual occurrence for me. I told Janet that my muscles were more clumsy today, probably because of the cold autumn wind. I began to wipe the coffee off using a paper napkin, which had been wrapped around plastic eating utensils, when I saw Steven's car screech to a stop. He ran to our table and stutteringly asked if I'd drunk or eaten anything. He ordered the other officers, who had just arrived, to secure the place for evidence, hurried us into his car, and sped to the safety of the campus police department.

It has been seven weeks since my brush with death. I find it ironic that my clumsy spastic muscles actually saved my life by delaying my first sip of coffee. The F.B.I. lab analysis showed a high amount of poison that would have certainly caused my heart to seize. The campus cops arrested Lazlow Price at the scene and charged him with two cases of murder in the first degree and one case of attempting to murder me. He is now in jail, being held there without bond. As I watch my students struggle with their final examination, I realize just how close death had been, and how the spilled coffee, and the time I had taken to clean it up, saved my life. Sometimes, just sometimes, being disabled is a blessing in disguise.

"Murphy's Inner World of Aphasia"*

He liked to be called "Murph," which was short for Murphy. Three years into retirement, he and Beth, his wife of forty-five years, were well-adjusted to the leisure life. Well, it was not exactly a life of leisure; the chores continued. Some days, it seemed retirement was more demanding and more active than the workaday world. If retirement was not the life of leisure Murph had always dreamed it would be, at least he set his own pace. And that meant a lot. Today was supposed to be a typical day in the world of the retired, and it was typical, except for one thing. In the next few hours, Murph's life would change forever. Murph would have a stroke.

The Great Cross-Country Journey was scheduled to begin next week. The pre-owned Bounder motor home had set them back a pretty penny, but what a great machine. Two televisions, a microwave, a CD player, and plenty of storage. Murphy would have preferred a diesel rather than the gas engine, but gas was relatively cheap. At seven miles to the gallon, it needed to be.

They had owned the machine two weeks, and Murph did not have buyer's remorse. In fact, he had buyer's glee over the best-looking recreational vehicle he'd ever seen, let alone owned. The Bounder had made Murph happier than he'd been in years. When Beth was out shopping, he would climb up into the driver's seat and just sit. Murph felt like he was on top of the world. He knew what people said about men and boys and the price of their toys. He also didn't care.

Murph knew he had a lot to do before embarking on the great adventure. The Bounder was in good shape but needed some TLC to be brought up to his high standards. Murph had always been a perfectionist. His son, Matt, had offered to help with the preparations, but Murph didn't like to impose on anyone, especially Matt. He knew Matt's twins were a handful, and his free time was limited, what with working overtime and all. The birth of the twins had stretched Matt's finances to the limit. Matt's wife, Andrea, had to return

*Reprinted by Permission: Tanner, D. (1999). The family guide to surviving stroke and communication disorders. Boston: Allyn & Bacon.

to work much too soon after the birth of Murph and Beth's only grandchildren. Murph felt a pang of guilt about spending so much money on the Bounder, but as they say in beer commercials, "You only go around once."

As Murph got into his pickup to go to the auto-parts store to buy road flares he hoped they would never need, a twinge of tightness gripped his right arm. For a moment, he could not open the door. The aging pickup had always had a sticky door, but this seemed unusual. "Oh well," he thought to himself, "I'll buy some oil for the hinges when I get to the store."

Driving to the store, Murphy tuned in to his favorite radio station. "The Country Voice of the Valley," they liked to proclaim. The nasal country tunes and the late morning sunshine made his increasing anxiety about the tightness in his arm dissolve. He had always liked country music. It was honest and all that. He couldn't imagine listening to anything else. As Murph pulled into the auto-parts store, the truck hit the curb with too much force. The jolt was enough to test the strength of the seat belt. "Damn," he thought, "There goes the front-end alignment. Now I'll have to get . . . to get . . . what's that called? . . ."

Murphy stepped out of the pickup and started walking to the entrance of the store. As he opened the door, again his right arm wouldn't do as he wanted. He stood there for a minute in confusion. "What's wrong with my arm?" he said to no one in particular.

On the way home, Murph was again at peace with the world. The guilt pangs about spending too much money on the Bounder still nudged at his conscience, but the confusion and anxiety slipped away. "Ah, the curative effects of country music," thought Murph.

Murph had always been one to ignore fear. He realized that during the war he had been more lucky than invincible and more lonely than fearful. Like most of his generation, the war had made him realize a lot. Whenever fear reared its ugly head, he was able to kick it back where it belonged. This method of coping had worked well throughout his life. Murph had the gift. If it bothers you, ignore it; it'll go away.

When Murphy got home, Beth was gone. She probably was visiting Matt, Andrea, and the twins. He didn't mind. He'd make one of his world-class sandwiches for lunch. Today, the sandwich would consist of three slices of ham, Swiss cheese, a dollop of horseradish sauce, a pickle, and a tad of mustard. There was no wheat bread, so he settled for the last two slices of white. Had Beth been home, she would have objected to the sandwich. She spent way too much time worrying about blood pressure, cholesterol, and salt intake. The sandwich was delicious, and as the last bite was swallowed, Beth walked through the door. That afternoon, Murph mentioned the problems with his arm and hand. He managed to work it into the conversation while complaining about the usual aches and pains. He minimized the event, more to protect himself from disturbing thoughts than to prevent her from overreacting.

Murph and Beth spent an uneventful evening together. After dinner, they talked about little things. She pretended to be interested in the playoffs, and he listened to more concerns about the grandchildren. There was a comfortable routine to their lives. It wasn't exciting, but it was predictable and secure. After the television was turned off, they retired to the bedroom. Murph's last words to Beth were, "Did you lock the doors?" As usual, he was asleep within minutes of his head hitting the pillow.

Murph was an early riser. It was hard for him to sleep when the sun was up. He had always considered himself a hard worker. Hard workers get up early, work hard, and go to bed tired. At 5:30 A.M., Murph opened his eyes. He felt the warm, comforting presence of Beth next to him. He heard the quiet snore, well, not a snore exactly, more of a muffled buzz. Beth was quite adamant about the fact that ladies do not snore. He quietly got up, always careful not to awaken his mate. If Murph was an early riser, Beth was the consummate nightowl. A lark married to an owl. Of course, Murph needed and always received that little catnap during the day. It was one of the perks of retirement. He silently planned the day's activities, careful to schedule that all important catnap. His biggest concern was a problem with the Bounder's air conditioning. "This could be an expensive day," he thought to himself.

As Murph walked toward the bathroom, he felt the strange sensation in his right arm again. His first reaction was one of irritation. He didn't have time for this nonsense. Only this time, it was not limited to his arm; the whole right side of his body felt strange. Suddenly, for the first time in a long time, Murphy was afraid. As Murph reached the bathroom door, his right side gave way, and he tumbled into the dresser. He tried to catch himself but to no avail. The family pictures carefully aligned on the dresser crashed to the floor, causing Beth to say, "What's wrong, Murph?" Murph didn't answer. He didn't understand the question. "Who's on?" he thought, what a strange thing for her to say.

Murph tried to get up, but it was no use. The entire right side of his body would not budge. Try as he would, Murph could not make his body move. Not his leg, arm, or hand. "This can't be happening," he thought. "What a strange dream," was his last coherent thought. Murph lost consciousness.

Beth was awakened by the startling early morning noise. Why would Murph knock the family pictures to the floor? It took only an instant for the events to register completely: Murphy was having a stroke. Maybe he was dying. She should have seen it coming. Strangely, Beth's immediate concern was the pictures on the floor and the broken glass. "Someone could get cut," she thought. Then she had the presence of mind to ask Murphy, "What's wrong?" There was no reply.

Beth dialed 911 on the bedroom telephone. "Nine, one, one. What's your emergency?" was the matter-of-fact voice on the other end. Within 20 minutes—20 long minutes—the paramedics arrived. The flashing lights woke the neighbors. There were sounds of police and ambulance radios. A stretcher was brought to the bedroom.

"It's clear the shush is," Murphy slurred. "He's delirious," thought Beth. She knelt down and tried to comfort him. Murph kept saying the strangest things. "It's shush, beyond." The utterances turned into unintelligible sounds and finally silence as Murphy gradually slipped into unconsciousness. Beth couldn't get the image of Murph lying on the bedroom floor out of her mind. It seemed so odd.

Beth saw the ambulance rush Murph off to the hospital. She was sure that this was just a minor and temporary problem. No way could this be happening to her. Murphy was too strong to fall victim to something like this. A feeling of calm surrounded her as she got into the car to drive to the hospital. There was relief in blotting from her mind the terrible things that were happening to her and Murphy.

Apparently, one of the neighbors had called Matt and Andrea. They met Beth at the hospital's main waiting room. It was good to see familiar faces. They hugged and talked grimly in low voices about the early morning shock. Beth was on the verge of tears. It was hard for her to stay in control. She was afraid of what this day would bring.

Murphy was brought into the emergency room. He became aware of the hustle and bustle, and it frightened him. It was too intense, too hectic. He was placed on heart, oxygen, and blood pressure monitors. Blood was taken for the lab tests, and oxygen tubes were placed in his nose. He was awake during most of the chaotic activities but had little understanding of what was happening. It was like a movie, a bad movie. A catheter was inserted to help with urination.

Twice, Murphy asked for Beth. Unfortunately, to the triage nurse it sounded like, "Care for mother." Murphy couldn't understand why the nurses, technicians, and doctors didn't seem to understand his perfectly normal speech. He then drifted into the sanctuary of sleep. Later that morning, Murphy had a vague sensation of claustrophobia while the CT (computerized axial tomography) brain scan was being conducted. He wanted to express his fear but was too tired to do so. He did not like being slid into the small tube. One thing bothered Murphy more than the claustrophobia—the shouting. Everyone felt the need to shout instructions. They would move their heads close to his ear and shout things Murphy was incapable of understanding. Apparently, they felt Murphy had lost his hearing.

Dr. William Tobbler, a board-certified neurologist, had been on call all night. It had been a long night; he had been called in to evaluate a youngster with a severe head injury. Seizure after seizure had shaken the little fellow's body. The seizures were finally under control, at least for now. As he watched the elderly man being wheeled into intensive care, he wondered if his services would be required. The man was pale, obviously paralyzed on the right side, and he heard the nurse say he couldn't communicate; he was aphasic.

He saw the hospital's oldest staff physician, John Foster, trailing after the new patient. John had his usual sour look and permanent frown plastered on his face. He liked Foster and the old-fashioned "country doctor" role he played. Watching him was like watching a rerun of *Marcus Welby, M.D.* John was considered a medical jack-of-all-trades.

The intensive care unit (ICU) is a strange place. Technology reigns supreme and the patients, the ones with the illnesses and injuries, appear to be an afterthought. The incessant beeping, clicking, and humming of the expensive machines are constant companions to staff and patients alike. In this hospital, there were 12 intensive care rooms. Murphy was placed in ICU-3. He lay on his back, a stiff sheet covering his body and a multitude of tubes and cords leading to and from him. The curtains were drawn, and the mute images of television flashed in the dimly lit room. Murphy had drifted in and out of sleep during most of the hours spent in the emergency room. He felt like an observer of the strange events occurring to him. It was easier to be an observer than a participant because it was all so unreal.

The first permanent memory Murph had of the ICU was the odor: disinfectant. There was no question in his mind that he was in a hospital; nothing smelled as clean and sterile as alcohol, and hospitals are drenched in it. Murph looked around. He recognized a few of the machines and most of the room's objects. He noted the tubes and lines attached to his body. He felt the irritation of the patches securing the sensors to his chest and arm. His mouth was dry and felt like cotton was stuffed in it. The oxygen tubes in his nose bothered him; he wanted to pull them out. Suddenly, panic gripped him; his hands were tied to the bed. He struggled, but it was no use. In hospital terminology, he was restrained, and restrained well. He couldn't scratch an itch if his life depended on it.

As Murph lay back, succumbing to the restraints, he felt calm; a sense of well-being surrounded him. As he stared at the hospital ceiling, he simply denied what had happened. He convinced himself that nothing bad was happening, and if it was, it wasn't happening to him. He welcomed the break from reality, and he slipped into the sanctuary of sleep.

When he awoke, Murph sensed he was in trouble. Something bad had happened. Hospital rooms like this were for people on the verge of death. From deep within his mind, thoughts of escaping from this dangerous place welled up. But strangely, he had no words to carry the thoughts. All that was present was the overwhelming need to escape. "Get me out of here!" was vocalized as nothing. No words came to his mind and no movements came to his lips. If Murph could have talked, he would have shouted: "I can't talk, help me!"

Beth met with Dr. Foster in the coffee shop. "It's serious, Beth," Dr. Foster pronounced. "He's had a serious stroke, and he might not make it. Even if he does pull through, his speech and ability to walk have been affected." This declaration was no surprise to Beth. She knew it was bad, and Dr. Foster had only confirmed it. A wave of sadness washed over her. It was the kind of feeling you get when a loved one is in serious trouble. Her first thought was to share this sad feeling with Murph. He'd understand the depth of it. He'd be strong.

Many doctors would have said to this anxious woman, "The CT scan showed an infarct in the left frontal region of the cortex, without a midline shift." Not Dr. John Foster. He had decided a long time ago that this type of medico jargon was a form of verbal abuse. He would never talk to family members, and especially his old friend Beth, like that. He simply said, "The X-ray showed damage on the left side of the brain, where speech is found. It is also the area that controls the right arm and leg. In fact, in Murph's case, the entire right side of his body may be paralyzed. It appears to be a clot and not a broken blood vessel."

Dr. Foster took the time to explain as much as he could to Beth.

"Yes, it's early.

"No, he's asleep now.

"Yes, his heart is strong.

"Yes, the stroke could get worse.

"No, brain cells do not grow back.

"No, he's not in a coma.

"Yes, he'll recognize you.

"No, he's not in physical pain."

"Our first goal is to get him stabilized, and then we'll begin thinking about rehabilitation," Dr. Foster planned aloud. He wanted to go into more detail but heard the beep of his pager. He checked the number and politely ended the conversation. As he walked off, Beth felt angry as the realities of the situation set in. She was angry with Dr. Foster for confirming the bad news and mad at herself for not doing something to prevent the stroke. She was also mad at Murphy for not taking better care of himself. All she could think was, "Why did this have to happen?" Beth was left alone in the crowded room, more alone than she had ever been.

Back in ICU, Murph saw Beth, Matt, and Andrea enter the room. Their grim faces triggered another bout of anxiety. He imagined their sad faces at his funeral. "Where are the twins?" he wondered in wordless thought. Their young, identical faces always brought a smile. Murph did not like the sad, forlorn faces on the three people he loved. He tried to say that it was all right and that things were going to be just fine, but there were no words, no sounds, no nothing. All that was present were images and sensations; there was no language to bring order to thought. He heard one and only one word surface to his mind's ear: "weird". As he attempted to verbalize it, nothing happened. As he tried again and again to express the weirdness of it all, his lips, tongue, and voice box suppressed it. The harder he tried, and the more force he brought to bear, the harder it was to command the movements of speech. With every increased effort to say, "w—eer—d," there was a corresponding increase in the resistance to program it. There were so few words he could remember, and when they did come to mind, they were too complicated to utter. Weird indeed.

Beth was careful not to disrupt the IV needle when she took Murph's hand. Her warm, firm hand in his was the first pleasant, comforting sensation Murph had experienced since his swan dive into the dresser. Tears swelled in his eyes and uncontrollable sobbing followed. Murph found himself crying like a baby. The crying was way out of proportion to the feelings he was experiencing. He wasn't that emotional or that sad. Talk about embarrassing. The nurse observing the family meeting made a mental note that Murphy was "emotionally labile." She had heard the doctors use that term to describe a patient who has exaggerated emotions due to brain damage.

Matt and Andrea were at a loss for words. They made small talk about the twins and other things, but it didn't take long for them to realize that the conversation was one sided. Murph saw the tears in Andrea's eyes, and once again, he cried. The embarrassment he felt was incredible. He tried to explain, but once again, all that came out was blathering nonsense. Murph had never felt so out of control, so utterly helpless. On a nonverbal level, he knew that if this was to be his future, death would be a welcome event.

As chance would have it, Dr. Tobbler arrived to consult on the patient in ICU-3 when Beth, Matt, and Andrea were there. He shook hands with the family and began to explain the medications Murphy was taking. The results of the CT scan were explained in frightening detail. Apparently, Murph was scheduled for an MRI—magnetic resonance imagery—test to further help pinpoint the site of the brain damage. Dr. Tobbler said that Murph's stroke was no longer in evolution, which Beth deduced was a good thing. It wouldn't get worse. In a day or two, Murph would be transferred to a regular hospital room.

Day two for Murph was as bad as day one. In fact, it was worse. The lunch tray was placed in front of him, and the nurse helped make the food manageable for a man with movement on only his left side. It was a puree diet, one obviously meant for stroke patients. Murph could barely manage the movement of the spoon to his mouth with his left hand, so a nurse's aide was sent in to help him. Murph knew the reputation of hospital food, but it did taste good. In fact, the smell, texture, and taste were welcome, familiar sensations. The nurse's aide was careful to keep the gray, brown, and yellow spoonfuls confined to the general area of his mouth. More embarrassment and more blows to his self-esteem. Murph had an image of himself as an ugly, overgrown baby with food smeared all over his mouth. But the real embarrassment was yet to come.

During the night, Murph's bowels moved. He felt the sensations and tried to call for the nurse but was unsuccessful. He knew he needed to call for a bedpan or to get up and go to the bathroom, but he didn't have the words to plan the acts. He wasn't confused; he knew what was going on. He was perplexed; he couldn't organize himself well enough to push the call light. He couldn't remember how to shout for the nurse.

He lay in his own waste, the smell overwhelming. On the most basic of levels, Murphy knew this was absolutely the worst thing that had ever happened to him. A kind nurse's aide came to his rescue. She cleaned him and the mess. Murph watched her face carefully for any indication of scorn or ridicule. None was detected and Murph was glad for that. There were few things to be glad about. As she was preparing to leave, Murph tried to utter something, anything, to lessen the embarrassment. Of course, even if he had been the most eloquent speaker in the world, nothing would have eased the awkwardness. Murph had the lowest image of himself he had ever had. The stroke had turned him into a babbling, drooling child, lying in his own waste. A little later, Beth entered the room and quietly sat down.

More words were becoming available to Murph. Fragments of complete inner statements occasionally came to mind. However, his verbal thoughts and visual imagery rarely connected. Occasionally, Murph understood the words of others. He had the most difficulty when people spoke rapidly or strung long sentences together. Dr. Foster asked him if he felt pain, and Murphy was convinced that the good doctor was informing him of the needed rain. Beth brought in a pencil and paper, hoping Murph could write his thoughts. Another blow to Murph's self-esteem: he wrote like a child. All he could muster were scribbles and a few lines that resembled his name. Everyone who saw the scribbles thought he was writing something profound. Matt saw the Bounder, Andrea saw the twins, and one nurse hurriedly brought him a bedpan. His writing was a makeshift inkblot test.

Dr. Linda Curzon was a 34-year-old physiatrist. She had been out of medical school only a few years, but she was more certain than ever that physical medicine and rehabilitation was the right specialty for her. She knew her trade and knew it well. The consult on the stroke patient in ICU-3 came early in the day. The attending physician was Dr. Foster. She'd had problems with Dr. Foster in the past. Old docs often tried to be one-man shows and resisted seeking her, or any other specialist's, opinion. She was director of rehabilitation and vice president of the medical staff, and it just might be that Dr. Foster was resentful of her age or specialty. That was his problem, she was a busy woman. She performed her usual thorough evaluation of rehabilitation potential on Murphy. There was a gleam in his eyes that she liked. The spark of life was still there.

During the course of her examination, Dr. Cruzon became angry. A tray had been ordered for this patient, and the nurses had eagerly fed the poor fellow. His face sagged, his tongue deviated on protrusion, his vocal cords would not close completely, and the gag reflex was absent. A first-year intern would have known that he was at risk for aspiration pneumonia. His temperature had spiked, and a person had to be deaf not to hear the gurgle in his lungs. Murph was sick and getting sicker. She placed him on NPO (nothing orally) status and ordered a chest X-ray, along with a speech and swallowing evaluation. She also ordered physical and occupational therapy. Her most pressing concerns were the swallowing problems and the potential for aspiration pneumonia.

Wendy, a certified speech-language pathologist, loved the interactions with the patients but hated the paperwork. The almighty paperwork. It wasn't even paperwork anymore, because the hospital had been computerized. All notes were entered into the central computer, and you had to request a printout to even see paperwork. Documentation, documentation, and more documentation. Sometimes she felt that she spent more time satisfying the needs of the bureaucrats and HMOs than the needs of the patients. As Wendy walked out of the therapy suite, the secretary pulled a slip of paper from Wendy's mailbox. Apparently, there was a new speech evaluation patient in ICU-3, a stroke patient of Dr. Foster's with aspiration pneumonia.

When Wendy walked into the ICU, she saw a nurse's aide leave the patient's room. The lingering odor spoke volumes of what had just happened. "The poor guy," Wendy thought. She said "hello" to one of the familiar faces in the unit and received a forced, obligatory nod. "They ought to rename this the insensitive care unit," Wendy thought as she typed her personal identification code into the unit's computer. Quickly, a complete history of the medical life and times of the patient was made available. She read his history, procedures, and consults with care. "Rather young to be losing so much," she thought. In her business, young was relative.

She walked into Murph's room and surveyed the situation. The woman sitting next to the bed was probably his wife, but Wendy had learned a long time ago not to make assumptions about relationships. Murph had his eyes closed, but she suspected he was not asleep. Many patients kept their eyes closed, especially after embarrassing events. It was a basic method of escape and avoidance. Gray thinning hair, thick eyebrows, and a bit on the heavy side, Murph was definitely the grandfather type.

Wendy greeted the woman seated next to the bed. She offered the details expected of her by providing her name and profession. She explained that her job was to evaluate Murph's speech, voice, language, and swallowing abilities. When that was completed, she would provide therapy to help the patient recover as much as possible. Beth had heard the same kind of speech from the physical and occupational therapists; only the names and faces changed. Wendy was careful to project both professionalism and empathy in the first contact. The negativity often associated with stokes could interfere with the working relationship if the clinician was not careful.

"Good afternoon" were the first words Wendy said to Murph. He opened his eyes and saw a young woman standing by his bed. He recognized the two words as a greeting but didn't know if she was bidding him good morning, good day, or good night. He smiled and nodded his head. Murph had already been stung too often with the pain of verbal impotence to attempt speech. Murph had learned quickly that it was a verbal crapshoot every time he opened his mouth. Occasionally he said the correct word, but more often than not, nothing came out or he blurted out the unexpected. Murphy sensed that this woman was responsible not for his blood, urine, walking, dressing, or breathing; she was here for his speech. He felt his first vague sense of hope.

Each time Murph tried to talk to Wendy, he fought to remember the word or struggled to program it. Even when he remembered the word and programmed it into existence, he produced it with a slur, a distortion caused by weak speech muscles. So far, all of his speech had been whispered. The familiar buzz of his voice box was absent. As Wendy tested his understanding of words, ability to sequence strings of sounds and syllables, and strength of speech muscles, Murph did his best to comply. After all, Murph had always been a hard worker and prided himself on that fact. Murph was glad that someone in the hospital understood the problems he was having with his speech. Wendy really understood, you could tell. She had seen other people adrift in this verbal confusion. Then Murph had another realization: he was not the only person who had ever had this problem. Wendy finished her evaluation and was talking to Beth about him. Beth nodded her head and asked questions. Occasionally, they both looked in Murph's direction.

Murph felt like a visitor in a strange, technologically advanced country. He didn't speak or understand the language of these foreigners. He recognized the objects, utensils, pictures, and uniforms as objects, utensils, pictures, and uniforms. The problem was that the names were different, or completely absent, in this strange foreign country. Most unusual.

The next morning, Murph was lifted from his bed to a wheelchair. He tried to help with the transfer but found that he was dead weight. So many times in his life he had gotten out of bed, and so often he had taken it for granted. He would never take easy movement for granted again.

As he was wheeled to the radiology section of the hospital, the people he passed in the halls and elevator greeted him in an uneasy manner. All he could do was nod his head and produce a slanted smile with his partially paralyzed face. He suspected that he looked a sight and wished they had combed his hair before leaving the room.

One of the signs on the entrance read "Nuclear Medicine", and Murph recognized and understood the word "Medicine." After a short wait in the X-ray room, yet another doctor, another specialist, introduced himself. The technicians lifted Murph from the wheelchair to the examining table and tilted him into a nearly vertical position. A long tube was pointed at his head and chest. Everyone dawned lead aprons, everyone but Murph that is. Again, Murph felt frightened. As he looked around, he saw Wendy enter the room. Her smile and friendly manner were comforting. To the technicians, Murph was 190 pounds of human mass to be held firmly in position. But to Wendy he was a person, an individual. At least, that was what Murphy sensed.

Liquid chalk; that's what it tasted like. The barium was a white substance swallowed while a video X-ray was taped. Wendy and the radiologist watched Murph, Murph's skeleton really, swallow the liquid. Most of it shot down into the stomach, but a small amount pooled on the vocal cords. When Murph took another breath, it went directly into his lungs. Murph did better with the barium paste and a cookie soaked in the stuff. But there was no question that Murph breathed the liquid. Wendy noted that, for now, Murph would not be able to eat or drink by mouth and that she would recommend that enteral, or tube feeding, be started.

The tube was coated with K-Y Jelly and slipped through his nose. The nurse kept telling Murphy to swallow. Actually, she was shouting the word. Once again, Murph wondered if there was something wrong with his hearing. Why would so many people feel the need to shout at him? His nose and throat hurt as the tube went down. Correction. Things don't hurt in a hospital; the patient feels some discomfort. Well, this discomfort hurt! When the end of the tube was finally resting in Murph's stomach and an X-ray was taken, the nurse started feeding Murph through the tube. A white liquid began to flow. This wasn't one of Murph's world-class sandwiches, but it was dinner. What was more important, it provided the needed liquids and protein. After a while Murph felt satisfied, not full, but satisfied.

The next day, Murph was moved to the intermediate care unit. In hospitalspeak, this is known as a step-down unit. It's not as intense as intensive care, but it's more intense than the acute floor. Murph was beginning to sense that there was a definite hierarchy in the hospital world.

Wendy and the other therapists visited him regularly in the intermediate unit. His right arm, leg, and hand were exercised, splinted, ultrasounded, and massaged. He was taught to stand, sit, and dress differently. Two days later, Murph was moved to the third-floor acute care ward. After learning to chew and swallow more carefully, the tube was pulled from his nose. What a wonderful sensation, almost as good as the taste of the soft food he was given. Soon after that, Murph was transferred to the rehabilitation section of the hospital. Murph knew something was up when Wendy jokingly said, "The vacation is over."

The fall that Murph had taken into the family pictures a few days ago seemed like a distant nightmare. Murph's life had changed permanently. From Murph's perspective, all of the changes were unwanted. In an instant, he was transformed into a dependent, verbally impaired patient in a large, impersonal institution. Although he could see and touch Beth, his mate of 45 years, a wedge had been driven between them. He still felt the love, the fondness for her, but all but the most basic expressions of his feelings were lost. Matt, Andrea, and the grandchildren visited him regularly, but there were painful silences and a lack of friendly chatter. He missed his old life sorely, and it angered him that so much had been taken from him. He certainly had not asked for the stroke, but he felt anger at himself for having it. He was angry at the whole situation. He was frustrated at being unable to change the situation, and that frustration also angered him.

The new relationships he had with the hospital staff were even less satisfying. Between exams, punctures, transfers, and drills, communication was a shadow of what it should have been. Murphy felt isolated, lonely, and depressed. Who wouldn't? His depression worsened as the reality of life after a stroke set in. The trigger, setting the depressive spiral in motion, was when Murph overheard that the Bounder was for sale. He couldn't understand the details, but it was clear from Beth and Matt's discussion that his Bounder was for sale. Murph slipped deeper and deeper into depression.

Some of Murph's speech and language had returned on its own. This was called spontaneous recovery. Within three weeks of the stroke, Murph's comprehension had returned to the extent that he could understand most of what was spoken to him, as long as people spoke clearly and slowly and avoided complex words. It irritated Murph that some people talked to him like he was retarded. He wasn't and didn't appreciate being talked to like that. It contributed to his depression. Murph could read short sentences and do some simple arithmetic problems. Each day he was getting better. Most patients who survive a stroke improve, at least somewhat. Words were still forced and slurred when he could find the correct ones, but his speech was now functional, which is hospitalspeak meaning he could express his wants and needs. Murph was able to write about as well as he could speak. Wendy told him this was typical for most stroke patients.

Wendy wanted Murph to be put on an antidepressant because he was too depressed, devastated by the recent events beyond a normal grief reaction. The injury to the cells of the brain and his inability to adjust to the unwanted events had combined to create a spiral of negativity. The poor guy just couldn't see the light at the end of the tunnel. Wendy would talk to Dr. Curzon about it.

The weekly rehabilitation meetings were highly structured, intense, and always interesting. The physiatrists ran the show and were quite democratic. Each doctor would provide a case history of the patient to be discussed and then call on the respective professionals for their ideas. Wendy sat quietly during the discussion of an 86-year-old woman with a fractured hip and diabetes. Murph was up next, and she wanted to make certain she covered everything in the brief time allotted to her.

Dr. Curzon matter-of-factly reviewed Murph's history. "The patient is a 68-year-old male who was transferred to the Rehabilitation Unit three days ago. He is stable and on antibiotics. The thrombosis interrupted blood flow of the middle cerebral artery to the left hemisphere. It was a relatively dense stroke. The patient had hemiparalysis, dysphagia, and was incontinent. He had aspiration pneumonia that is now under control and responding well to the medications."

The physical therapist reported that Murph was doing well. He was still at an "assist level," meaning that he was far from being able to walk by himself. Murphy was having trouble transferring from bed to wheelchair and back again. Wendy was delighted to hear that some movement was returning to Murph's right hand. She recalled the lecture from long ago in which the professor reported that speech recovery often correlates to the return of function in the right hand.

The occupational therapist reported that Murph was unable to dress himself but was learning self-sufficiency at the expected rate. She noted that Murph was not very motivated lately. She explained how Velcro was substituted for zippers and buttons and that Murph was improving in other ADLs. Activities of daily living were always called ADLs. Wendy was impressed with the tricks of the trade the occupational therapists had. They were quite clever in teaching patients alternate ways of dressing and eating.

The report from the dietician was relatively standard for a stroke patient. Wendy often chuckled to herself when the dietician reported that a particular patient was 10 to 15 pounds over his or her ideal weight. "Who wasn't?" she thought.

The social worker reported that Murph's finances were good. He was in a designated Medicare bed and had supplemental insurance. Out-of-pocket expenses would still be considerable, but apparently the family resources could handle it. She noted that Beth was a concerned, caring spouse and was adjusting well to Murph's disabilities. As an aside, she reported that Matt tended to be too protective and somewhat anxious about his father. The social worker's final statement was a good introduction to Wendy's presentation. She said that Murphy was depressed and becoming more so.

Wendy reviewed Murph's swallowing status. He was on a soft diet and tolerating it well. As long as he took a deep breath before each swallow and paced himself, there were no occurrences of choking or coughing. She was going to advance his diet and stop the Thick-it. Thick-it was a substance put in the patient's liquids to provide more texture. It helped the patient manage thin liquids during swallowing. Thin liquids, such as juices and coffee, tended to be the most difficult items for the patient with swallowing problems.

Wendy noted that Murph's receptive abilities had improved considerably since her first visit to him in ICU. She reported the results of the Token Test, in which the patient follows commands by pointing to or rearranging differently colored and shaped objects. "Murph can understand the majority of speech. Writing seems to be the modality of communication least improving," she reported.

Wendy noted that programming of the words seemed to be the main difficulty. "Murph," she reported, "has more problems sequencing and planning the utterances than he does in retrieving the words." Both finding the correct name and then being able to plan and program it into existence were problematic. This was the nature of his type of aphasia. She condensed it into the professional jargon everyone at the conference table would understand: "The patient has Broca's aphasia with a predominance of apraxia of speech. He also has mild dysarthria."

Wendy then asked Dr. Curzon if she would consider prescribing an antidepressant for Murphy. She stated that he was extremely depressed, and it was not resolving on its own. She was also concerned at his listlessness and lack of motivation. She thought the antidepressant would help increase his motivation and his ability to benefit from therapy. That was the professional rationale provided to Dr. Curzon. Wendy knew the main reason was that Murph was in pain—psychological pain—and it hurt her to see him suffer. In a few days, the antidepressant would kick in and Murph's spirits would elevate. Then, along with the return of more function, he would likely find the strength to adjust to his communication disorders. Too much had gone wrong in this guy's life, too much, too rapidly. Antidepressants provided many patients a leg up on the adjustment process. As a psychologist once told the staff at a rehabilitation meeting, "It's hard to learn to navigate in a storm. The medications calm the seas."

Wendy had been right—the time spent in ICU, intermediate, and acute care was a vacation compared to the rehabilitation ward. Everything was structured from morning to night. He was dressed and ready to go by 7:15 A.M. Breakfast was usually taken in his room, although lunch and dinner were held in the communal dinning room. By 8:30 A.M., Murph was in the physical therapy gym learning to walk with the assistance of a walker. Things were not going well with the walker. He just couldn't keep his balance. If it weren't for the help of the aide, he would have fallen more than once. Occupational therapy was helping him become more independent in dressing and feeding himself. He was learning to transfer from his wheelchair to the toilet without falling.

Murph had therapy with Wendy twice a day. He eagerly anticipated the morning and afternoon sessions. The exercises, drills, and games were helping him to remember words and ease their production. His facial muscles were becoming stronger, his speech was more precise. The most difficult hurdle to overcome was the tendency of his mouth to have a mind of its own. Some sequences of sounds and certain words were unavailable to him. Try as he would, he just couldn't get the sounds to come out correctly.

"Automatic speech" was a strange phenomenon. Some words and phrases were impossible to speak when he tried to do so. However, when his mind was elsewhere and he wasn't trying to force speech, those words and phrases were spoken easily and articulately. His daughter-in-law's name was a good example. Once in the morning session, Murph was trying to say her name. As he practiced her name, all that came out was "dan rea," "san vea," "dorn a hea." The harder he tried, the more thought he put into it, the further he got from the word. Then, as if in some bizarre magic show, he turned to Wendy and said, "Can't seem to say Andrea today." The automatic utterances were quite frequent and, much to Murph's dismay, readily present on swear words. Murph had never been one to swear much. He was not a crude man. But, boy, the swear words were easy to say since the stroke. They would pop out at the worst times, too. He had to work to forget the first words he accidentally said to the minister during his visit. In some ways, automatic speech was a curse.

Wendy had prepared Murph for group. She had managed to explain to him that he was going to be provided therapy at the same time as some of the other patients. She wheeled Murphy into the large room and placed the locks on the wheelchair when he was in position at the table.

Across from Murph sat a young man. His head had been shaved and a curious question mark scar was prominent next to his ear. Murph said, "Good morning. My name is Murphy." Actually, Murph said, "Should morning . . . name, Murph." He wanted to correct the errors, but Wendy had been clear that the best strategy was to keep going forward in these situations. Too many patients spent too much time revising and correcting, struggling and fighting to make the output perfect. In the world of aphasia, perfection is rarely attainable. She was right. The question mark kid had understood what Murph said and replied in a slurred, distorted way.

To Murphy's left was another man. He was about Murph's age. Like Murphy, his arm was also secured to his chest. He nodded when they made eye contact and burst into tears. Murphy knew what was happening; he'd been there, done that. In fact, he was still there, still doing that as he fought to stop his own tears.

Across from the crying man was a woman in her mid-50s. She was a pleasant looking woman who smiled at Murph and said, "Hello, my name is Helen. Welcome to our kroop, stroop." She then opened her mouth widely and carefully said, "group." Murph nodded.

Next to the woman was another man, clearly older than anyone at the table. He just stared out the window; he didn't acknowledge anyone or anything. He had a blanket wrapped around him, and a tube was running from his nose up to a plastic bag that hung on a steel hanger attached to his wheelchair.

Another man walked into the room. At first Murph thought he might be one of the doctors. He waved and nodded to everyone at the table, then turned to Wendy and precisely said, "The chitters have arranged." Now Murph was still having a problem understanding the speech of others, but this was clearly an odd thing for anyone to say. Then the man turned to Murph and followed his observation about the chitters with the statement,

"A new chit. Gone a hafta depend on it?" Then the man looked directly into Murph's eyes and awaited a response.

Murph heard a strange sound coming from his throat. It had been a long time since he had last heard it. He was laughing, laughing out loud. It wasn't Murphy's style to laugh at other people, but this was just too funny. He looked around and all of the patients, except the man in the blanket, were laughing. Wendy seemed to enjoy it the most. When the laughter subsided, Wendy carefully explained to Murph that Mr. Skinner had jargon aphasia. Apparently, the understanding centers of his brain were damaged, and he had a degree of denial about the communication disorder. Mr. Skinner believed that he was talking normally and that people just needed to take the time to understand him. Murphy had a vague recollection of experiencing a similar feeling in the emergency room.

Murph looked forward to group. As time passed, he became friends with Mr. Skinner and the question mark kid. He met the pretty woman's family and tried to build a bridge to the blanket man. But the blanket man was too distant, too alone. Murph hoped he would come around and some-day become a participant in group. Murphy learned to accept the group members for what they were, for what they had become. They were all travelers on a difficult road. They all had lost so much. But they were all gaining, too. New friends, new skills.

Beth helped Murph into the old pickup. He noted that she had trouble opening the door. He'd have to remember to get some oil for the hinges. With the wheelchair in the back, they drove to their home of 40 years. It was good to be home. He had forgotten how pleasant and predictable a home could be. He managed to get around, mostly in the wheelchair. Matt had made the house wheel-chair accessible by building ramps and making two doors wider. Murph still saw Wendy for outpatient therapy three times a week, but at least he was home. Although his speech was far from perfect, he got by. Each day more words came to him. Just like before the fall into the dresser, each new day was an unknown. There would be the good and the bad, the positive and the negative. The stroke had changed many things, but the days continued.

Beth watched Murph playing with the twins in the yard. Murph would count, and the twins would run from the fence to a tree. She enjoyed hearing the laughter and the screams from the twins. She thought about the Bounder and the trip they would never take. Her thoughts about the motor home and the Great Cross-Country Journey were interrupted by the sight of the twins, both of them, hugging their grandpa. Murph was home.

"Alternately Abled"

Chapter One

Sometimes you misjudge people. It is so easy to jump to conclusions, so comfortable to rely on tried and true stereotypes, no matter how untested they are. Prejudices are natural, you know. We "pre-judge." When sitting on a chair, you know it will hold your weight because, in the past, thousands of chairs have saved your butt from crashing to the floor. You expect the sun to rise in the morning because it has peeked over the horizon every day since there were eyes to witness the explosion of light and color. You pre-judge your car's stopping power on icy roads, the wince and watery eyes of too many drops of Tabasco sauce, and the certainty that your dog will keep running even when you demand its halt. You are unconsciously certain that electrons will reach the bulb when you grope for the light switch early in the morning; they will because they have. We must pre-judge; our sanity relies on it. The world would be a frighteningly chaotic blur if the past did not foretell the future.

It is our prejudices about people that muck up the works. Two rude blond waitresses and you expect the third to be surly. A criminal markup of parts and labor by one mechanic and you expect the same from all grease monkeys. Being mugged by a young man with baggy pants and tattoos of snakes alerts your nighttime senses to all males, loose-fitting pants and reptilian body art. Prejudices about people are the same type of generalization, the same process of predicting the future, but sometimes they are fraught with error.

I did everything I could to keep the Cessna in the air, to keep it flying. From the time I heard the sickening clunk and grinding of pistons and bearings gone awry, I went by the book. In the world of aviation, every eventuality has been anticipated, and there are rules for dealing with them. That's what "flying by the book" means. I tried to restart the engine. Three times I tried to get the propeller to turn, but it seemed frozen—super-glued in place. The only sound was the whoosh of the air as the dead plane began to drop from the sky. The passengers were quiet and frozen like the plane's engine. I looked for a flat, smooth place to land, but Alaska is a rugged place. The river, winding through the deep canyon, seemed the least of the landing evils. A water landing would be bad but not nearly as disastrous as shooting through pine trees.

Yes, I was frightened, but there was little time and too much to do to be consumed by fear. I knew I would do my best and, with luck, save my life and the lives of my passengers. As the trees and river rapidly approached, I shut off the fuel. In the microphone of my Sony headset, I announced our impending doom to anyone and everyone. On the emergency band, I declared every pilot's worst fear: "Cessna three four four five niner, May Day, May Day. Lost power, crash landing into Dolores River. Cessna three four four five niner, May Day, May Day." I heard some whimpering and quiet sobbing from the passengers, but much to their merit, there was no panic, no shouting, no screaming. I told them to tighten their seat belts and shoulder harnesses, to cover their faces with their hands, and to get out of the plane as soon as possible when we were in the water. I also said we were going to make it; we were going to walk away from this landing. Little did they know that it was said more for my benefit than theirs.

We were a long way from anyone. Alaska can be desolate. I knew that even if we survived the landing, getting home would be an equally challenging feat. "Cessna three four four five niner, May Day, May Day. Lost power, crash landing into Dolores River." I then "squawked" my identification by pressing 34459 on my instrument panel, hoping it would light up our position, speed, direction, and other valuable information on the Fairbanks tower's radar screen. "Cessna three four four five niner, May Day, May Day. I'm about 130 miles north, northeast of Tuktoyucktuk. Cessna three four four five niner, May Day, May Day."

Gravity continued to pull us down until I could clearly see the pinecones hanging from the tops of the trees. I fought the reflex to pull back on the yoke and try to make the airplane climb from the approaching danger. I kept the nose down and the speed up. I aimed for the smoothest part of the choppy river and shouted "Hang on, brace yourselves" to the passengers. I turned the main power switch to off. Then, a calm fell over me. It is the kind of feeling you get when you realize that you've done your best and everything is now in the hands of God and fate. There are no more decisions, no more options. Life and death will play out, and I was just an observer to the unfolding events. About ten feet above the water, I pulled up the nose of the plane and tried for a controlled stall, so as to stop in midair, and gently drop to safety.

Unbelievably cold. The water was freezing cold and it numbed my senses. I was disoriented. I couldn't tell up from down. I swallowed and choked on cold, blood-soaked Alaskan water. My lungs ached and demanded oxygen. Something twisted and red pinned my right leg, and I couldn't free it. I was flailing, struggling to free myself, but I really wasn't panicked. I was resigned to my watery fate and the struggle was just an act, something my body needed to do. All I could hear was the muffled roar of the river. Just as I started to lose consciousness, I felt two strong hands tug, jerk, and pull my pinned leg. There was a little movement, then more, and finally I broke free from the death grip. Those same strong hands grabbed the lapels of my flight jacket and pulled me through the small crumpled door of the Cessna. Through the cold, clear Alaskan water, I could see a round face wince as he struggled to push me to the surface. My rescuer was the heavyset one. My lifesaver was one of the passengers. As I broke through the surface of the river and sucked in the wonderful fresh

Alaskan air, I realized I had been saved by one of the retarded passengers. My savior was one of them that I had dismissed, felt superior to, and made jokes about. He was the good-natured one. I owed my life to him. He had risked his own life, dove beneath the surface, forced himself through the small opening, and freed my leg. And he did it with four broken ribs and a nasty slash on his shoulder and back. Sometimes you misjudge people.

Chapter Two

I love this campus. Hundreds of grassy green acres dotted by huge oak and maple trees, flowering bushes, and small manicured gardens. Thousands of students swarm this academic sanctuary, busily rushing from one class to another, to and from the library complex, and home to dingy dorm and apartment. Sometimes I sit on one of the iron benches outside the International Center and just take in the sights, sounds, smells and energy that is this large Midwestern university. I study the young and not-so-young men and women confidently pursuing their studies with the hope that their future will be better because of it. It's called "delayed gratification." It is the act of putting off house, Corvette, garden, profession, and family until the four, six, or eight years of study are complete. It's the belief that all will work out for the best and those years of timed tests, teaching, and tutoring will pay off. It is the belief that the pay will be not just in money, but also in quality of life. Higher education is a promise our society makes to the intelligent. And usually the promise is fulfilled. Education is good.

There are so many different types of people soaking up the rich education this campus has to offer. Bearded young men with very intense faces, jocks with fancy cars and bruised bodies, granolas and tree huggers, sorority sisters, stoners, young republicans, cowboys, and debaters. There are thespians, always on stage and making grand entrances, medical students haughtily burdened by huge books on pathology and pediatrics, future lawyers planning and scheming to get the biggest slice of the American pie, aspiring accountants, psychologists, and managers. I know I should be sent to a nauseating sexual harassment workshop, but I enjoy watching the women. I watch them walk, sit, smile, and be. As I ride this diesel coughing bus to my office, I study them. I particularly like women who wear glasses. I wonder about their hot, sensual ways hidden behind their librarian facade. She just smiled at me, eyes sparkling, legs crossed, breasts present. It sends my heart into arrhythmia, and I can feel the blood rush to my face.

Of course, my thoughts of her are pure fantasy with nary the slightest chance of becoming reality. You see, I'm a gimp. Cerebral palsy has given me the walk and talk of a pitiful person. I have these crutches that help me get from here to there, but I'm clumsy, awkward, and slow. I have spastic muscles constantly fighting and pulling against each other. My voice is raspy and my speech is slow. It seems I'm constantly repeating myself to the "What," "Pardon," and "Huh" of my listeners. It gets frustrating and sometimes downright infuriating. I know I have a good mind. I am a professor, after all, with diplomas and an academic gown to prove it. I was told by my high-school sweetheart that I also have a good personality. If the sensual librarians would get to know me, they would see I am passionate about my passions, quick-witted, and thoughtful. I've got a great imagination, probably because I need one. So many things are out of reach for me physically, but I can soar in my mind. In my mind, the sweet, sensual librarian is lying exhausted on the sweat-soaked bed, flush-faced, begging me to return as I dress, look for my car keys, and hurry off to my 10:00 A.M. course. Thank God for an imagination and women who wear glasses.

I must keep my fantasy flights about librarians secret. If I were normal physically, I suppose some women would find them a turn-on. If I were normal physically, most men would chuckle, realizing that this is how real men think. It's a guy thing and the politically correct might just as well try to stop the wind from blowing as to bring an end to these fantasy romps. But, as a gimp with slow and awkward speech, I better keep them to myself. For normal men, the fantasies are as natural as breathing, but for me, they're a perversion. Sex and the disabled are taboo. It's something about the gene pool and propagating the best and fittest. I sure as hell better keep my flights of fantasy a secret from my girlfriend, Janet. I'd be looking for more than my car keys if I shared my librarian secrets with her.

The closest bus stop to my office is about a thousand feet away. A thousand feet doesn't seem like much to someone with strong legs and a normal body, but for me it's a challenge, especially when there are snow and ice to deal with. We had a late spring snow about a week ago, and there are still ice spots dotting the sidewalk. After the bus pulled away and the cloud of diesel lifted, I began my shuffle. First, the metal cane attached to my right-hand finds a secure spot, then I shift my weight to it, and drag and slide forward. Next, my left hand performs the same act of locomotion and off I go, the strain of each step showing on my face. Plop-slide, plop-slide, plop-slide. Hundreds of students and a fat, bearded colleague float by me, not making eye-contact and hurrying to their destinations. A thousand feet is about three football fields, and like a star halfback, I go from goal to goal dodging people and things while the crowd cheers. When I get to the door of the Arts and Science Annex, I must push the large blue handicapped button for it to open. Today a middle-aged woman, tall and slender, smiles at me and pulls it open. She has large, dark eyes, darker skin, and very short hair, showing off her long, sensual neck. I like long, sensual necks. As I plop and slide through the opened door, I detect a wisp of strawberry or sage. I slur a "thank you" and muster a smile at her kindness. Several students stand to the side, allowing me enough room to park a semi. As I continue forward on the gray and white checkered tile, I hear her whisper a loving, adoring song: "Be careful Ben. I'll wait forever if necessary." Then, as I bravely begin the rescue of the children, assault rifle strapped to my strong back and determination on my rugged, handsome face, I hear her shout, "I love you." Dramatic marching music plays in my ear as I risk life and limb for the children held by the evil terrorists. "We need to talk." In an abrupt flash, I am jolted back to reality by the sound of Janet's voice. I see her sitting on a chair next to my office door.

Janet and I have been together for seven years. The more time I spend with her the more I love her. She's intelligent, beautiful, and compassionate. She has long, jet black hair and her skin is fair and smooth. She has the kind of smile that brightens up the darkest room, and you can get lost in her eyes. When she looks at you, her eyes burn to the very core of your soul. I've never had the courage to ask her why she chose to be with me, what with all the normal, handsome men in the world, preening and strutting for her attention. And she could have any of them. I've seen their eyes follow her as she walked down a hall or out of a room. Physically, she's like a magnet, and her personality is even more seductive. The closest I have come to understanding her willingness to be with me was when I asked her why she chose to work with the disabled. After all, she could be a smartly dressed executive, lunching and planning corporate policy with smartly dressed subordinates who hang on her every word. In the corporate world, she could have had all of the trappings of power, money, and success. But the path she took is cluttered with concrete thinking, drooling, seizures, acting out, slurred speech, and frustration. Her answer to my question was, typically, to the point: "It's just what I do." As best as I can tell, Janet has only one flaw; she has a blind spot. She doesn't see us as defective or deficient. She takes us at face value.

I keep my office tidy. It's not that I am a tidy person, it is just that ambient junk can cause a gimp like me to fall to the hard floor. So, I'm a tidy person by necessity, not by an ordered mind. Janet sat on the small couch donated to the Center where she works. I bought it for $20.00, and it was delivered by Elroy and Nick, two of the strongest residents at the Center. Both have Down syndrome and are in their twenties. I like them both, but I like Elroy the most. Elroy is a very thoughtful person, in his own way. I know he has the hots for Janet and he does little to hide it. When he is around her he blushes, fumbles, and befuddles. He adores her, as do I. I've resolved that if he gets any more bold with her, I might have to kick his befuddled butt. That would be a sight, he and me fighting for the hand of the Damsel.

"They funded it. The grant came through," Janet announced with that soft, sensual voice that turns me to jelly. About a year ago, she applied for a grant from a private foundation for a field trip for some of the residents of the Center. According to excited Janet, Horizons, a privately held philanthropic organization, funded, in total, the trip to Alaska. Five members of the Center and Janet and I would jet to Anchorage and then to Fairbanks. Then, a bush pilot would fly us to a fishing and hunting cabin where we would experience the great outdoors in order to develop character and independence. When she was writing the grant, I thought the whole idea was crazy. What organization in its right mind would donate, with no strings attached, the thousands of dollars necessary for a wilderness trip for a bunch of defectives? Apparently Horizons did and they didn't bat an eye. Thanks to Horizons, we would have this great Alaskan adventure.

The Center for Human Development is located west of the university on State Street. The Center is made of red brick, with window and door frames painted white. Actually, there are three buildings and a grassy green area the residents call the "park." The administrative building is the smallest of the three structures but has the finest office equipment, carpet, and furniture. The dormitory building consists of sixteen apartments, each specially designed for mentally and physically impaired dwellers. There is also a dining room in the basement. The industrial shop and retail store are where business is conducted. People can purchase donated furniture, clothing, lamps, toys, office equipment, small and large appliances, books, and a host of other discarded, tax deductible items in the store. All of the goods are sorted, cleaned, repaired, and made presentable by the mentally and physically defective residents and supervisors of the facility. Those with the lowest I.Q.s sort and hang clothing. The ones with higher but still defective minds do various other tasks to make the goods sellable. The Center also contracts with apartment buildings and businesses to clean and manicure their grounds. Some of the residents have regular eight-to-five jobs and are hustled off every morning to coffee shops, restaurants, and industrial parks in a white stretch van with the Center's name proudly painted on the doors. Janet is Director of Vocational Services and is loved by everyone at the Center, especially Elroy.

Chapter Three

Lunch break at the Center is like free time at any blue-collar place of employment. Some of the women sit at a table, talk, and eat from brown bags. Other workers lie on soft bundles of clothing, sleeping or just resting their eyes. A young couple eats together in a secluded corner of the lounge making small talk, laughing, and planning their future. A radio blasts tunes in the warehouse while several young men play touch football. Elroy crouches behind a center grunting "Hut one, hut two, hut three" and finally takes the ball from a man who has no idea what a "hut" or a "three" is. Elroy drops back, plants his feet firmly, and throws a short pass to a 30-year-old man with a mental age of eight. He manages to catch the ball but is immediately tagged by a buck-toothed line backer with a serious drooling problem. Don't most linebackers have drooling problems? Two college women, dawning the first skimpy shorts of spring, walk past the large warehouse doors between the two parked trucks, and "time" is called. The football players watch them meander down the sidewalk, and a few men make the comments heard at most construction sites by burley hardhats who think a catcall is the same as foreplay. Has any woman ever stopped, walked back to the hardhats and found them irresistible? Lunch break at the Center is like free time at any blue-collar place of employment.

Elroy watches Ben and Janet enter the administrative offices. Seeing Janet brightens his day. Immediately, he calls an end to the ball game and walks toward the administration building. The players with quizzical looks on their faces mill around, wondering what happens next. Elroy's mind quickly conjures a reason to talk to her. Of course his motives are transparent to all with I.Q.s above seventy. All Elroy is aware of is the pressing need to hear her voice, see her smile and maybe, just maybe, be touched by her soft, warm, feminine hands. She often grasps his arm or strokes his shoulder when discussing his phoney, made-up topics. Actually, Elroy isn't much more awkward than most ten-year-old males with a crush on an older woman. After all, Elroy really is just a ten-year-old in a body that has aged twenty-six years.

"Do we lock up?" Elroy asks as he stands too close to her. Janet immediately stops walking and smiles, "Of course, but not now, Elroy." Had Elroy a tail, it would have wagged. He looked at Ben and snortingly said, "Not now." In Elroy's world, he had taken Janet away from his rival and, through shear cunning, won the competition for her heart. She was now with him, torn away from Ben. Her warmth was all his and he lorded it over Ben. His grin and eye-contact clearly said, "Take that, Professor." In the world of sub-average I.Q.s, Janet had chosen him and the relationship would last forever. Score one for the home team.

In the conference room, Janet made the announcement to the five lucky residents. Four of them, and Ben, sat on steel folding chairs. Elroy sat next to Janet, on the edge of a conference table, basking in her warmth, clearly the dominant male with his prize. Next to Ben was Anastasia. Her life at the Center began with her mother's drinking problem. Anastasia's case history said her mother had died of alcoholism in her mid-forties. Actually, the cause of death was listed as an automobile accident late one Saturday night. But her death was really caused by wine coolers and scotch chasers. She was a binge drunk and, during one of them Anastasia was born. For eight months before her birth, Anastasia developed in an alcohol-saturated womb. It left her frail, frightened, and mentally deficient. Even now, as she approached nineteen, Anastasia's life was a hangover. When she reached out, which was not often, Anastasia spoke slowly and rarely understood complicated instructions. She was also prone to temper tantrums. She worked at the most menial jobs, the ones that required the least of her deficient problem-solving abilities. Anastasia's job at the Center was to sort hangars. She saw to it that wire, blue, yellow, and white hangers were placed with their own kind.

Autism wreaked havoc on his young parents eighteen years ago, but Rusty appeared normal at first. He nursed, crawled, and cried like most babies. His mother, an only child herself, thought all was well until nagging suspicions were confirmed by specialists. As Rusty grew to be a toddler, he became more distant and aloof. Often, he treated his loving parents as objects in the same detached manner as he did his mechanical toys. But it was the echolalia that frightened them. Most normal children go through a stage of speech development where they repeat what has been spoken. But Rusty did it all of the time and never outgrew it. He also liked to see the light flicker when he strobed his fingers close to his eyes. Echoed speech, hand stimulation, and a tendency to rock back and forth had led to Rusty's life at the Center. It was all too much for the loving parents, and when their marriage collapsed Rusty had nowhere to go. But he was soon to go to Alaska and experience the great outdoors and, perhaps, find an escape from his shell.

The other two adventurers were becoming an item at the Center. Trevor and Nicole, both seventeen, were feeling the teenage chemistry. They both had a fondness for fruit punch, and it was at the soft-drink machine where they began. Trevor was borderline in his intelligence and had the endearing manner of Forrest Gump. Nicole had fallen head-over-heals in love with him. Trevor had begun to return her love, but it was taking time. It simply took more time for Trevor to process life. He wasn't put off by her deformed back and legs. In fact, he found her physically irresistible, especially her young breasts. They mesmerized him. Two weeks ago, she had let him touch them. After "lights out," she had quietly knocked at his apartment door, and they had slipped to the basement and found the large linen closet unlocked and inviting. Nothing was said as she removed her blouse and unfastened her bra. She took his hands and, for the first time, Trevor touched them. Electricity shot through their bodies as they kissed and caressed. Body heat rose and rapid breathing was all that was heard. There was an uncontrollable, primal need to be closer, to be one. But a car's alarm system frightened the young lovers and abruptly ended the passion. Coming from the staff parking lot, the honk, honk, honk brought an early end to their exploration. They returned to their respective floors without being caught, determined that there would be a next time—and soon. That night, they both lay on their beds reliving the passion, their hearts resonating with the intensity of young love.

Chapter Four

Autumn is my favorite season, but spring ranks second. In spring, trees return to life, flowers bloom, grass turns green, and the days get longer. I need longer days. I need sunshine. I get moody and depressed during the winter when the days are short and the sky is overcast. In the dark, dreary months of winter, my problems seem bigger, my frustrations greater, and my cerebral palsy more handicapping. I just don't feel good. I eagerly anticipate Spring Break. For many of the students on this campus, Spring Break is a long car ride to Florida, Mexico, or Arizona, beer, and one-night-stands. But for me, Spring Break signals the end of the wintry dark and the brightness of renewal.

I've done the Spring Break ritual once, but I seemed to be an observer rather than a participant. My buddies were good about helping me get around, finding plenty of room for my crutches, and listening politely while I droned on. But they won the girls, drank the beer, and puked the poison from their bodies over the balcony of the motel room. They spent the night in the drunk tank and barely remembered the brawl. Oh, I wanted to win the girls, but with so many tanned, normal male bodies available it just wasn't in the cards. What woman would want to boast of a romp with a gimp? How seductive can you be with spastic speech? I drank a few beers, but I'm tipsy enough without them. Besides, I have to be careful with alcohol because the more I drink, the less disabled I am. After a six-pack or so I'm Superman but much more handsome and with a wonderful ability to sing. In fact, I sang "Buh, Buh, Bad to the Bone" while my buddies brawled. Well, someone had to.

I teach literature. It is my calling in life. When I lecture to large classrooms of students, sometimes I lose myself in Hemingway, Steinbeck, Grafton, Hillerman, and MacDonald. I may be physically imperfect, slow of speech, and clumsy of body, but when my mind is saturated with literature, I become one with its glory and perfection. Sometimes students sense my rapture and join me in the depth of thought that is literature. I love it. I even like reading their papers. Oh, I know most have only read the Cliff's Notes, but every now and then a sophomore from a farming community or a tenement in the projects will connect with a great writer's mind and story. She will sense the writer's marvelous ability to turn a phrase and, in turn, capture something profound about the human condition. Then, she too, will turn a phase, sometimes as eloquent as the writer's and teleport those insights to me in the form of a twelve-page paper, double-spaced and carefully spell-checked. Unfortunately, with scores of papers to grade, I can only note my pleasure at her growth with a brief statement made with red ink, apply an "A" to her new and hard-fought insights and move onto the next paper in the foot-high stack.

Spring term rolled along, and as the great Alaskan adventure approached, both Janet and I began to plan for the trip. It's true that the Devil, not God, is in the details. Tickets were purchased, and the airline was told of the special needs of its passengers. Permission forms were completed by parents and guardians, and boots and raincoats were purchased. Hours were spent on the telephone to Anchorage, Fairbanks, and bush pilots. The weather channel was watched intensely to see what was typical for that part of the huge state of Alaska. Several times Janet and I both confessed that we may have bitten off more than can be chewed. The Alaskan adventure would bring out the best and worst of all of us. It would test our mettle.

Chapter Five

Watching them laugh, share bites of sandwiches and chocolate bars, and touch each other's arms and thighs, Janet knew the time had come. Nicole and Trevor had moved to the next level, and things needed to be done. Birth control was going to be necessary, and perhaps it was already too late. Janet was matter-of-fact about these things. It wasn't a question of morality, it was one of reality. Janet was not a fuddy-duddy. The reality was that without birth control soon Nicole and Trevor would bring another life into this world. Not that there was anything wrong with that; they had every right, even a biological obligation, to begin their lives together and to have children. It was simply a matter of timing and choice. They were both too young, and for them, because of their disabilities, special plans needed to be made before they jumped into the rest of their lives and the responsibilities of a new one. Things needed to be thought out and not left to chance and the back seat of a car. Janet and Melissa, another counselor at the Center, would take the initiative, make the appointments, and do the counseling. All of this had to be done quietly, almost secretively. People don't like the idea of sex and the disabled. It makes them uncomfortable. It makes some people ugly.

Janet had been with the Center for twelve years. It was her first professional job since graduating from the university with a master's in rehabilitation counseling. Her primary job was to find employment for residents of the Center. She had been very lucky. She had also been very persuasive in showing their abilities rather than their disabilities. Some of them worked in the auto parts plant sorting nuts, bolts, and screws and placing them in small plastic packages. Some bussed tables, mopped floors, and placed dirty dishes in washing machines. One of the residents, a middle-aged man with many disabilities including deafness, worked next to a noisy industrial mixer while it ground and combined rocks and chemicals. Prolonged noise exposure was not a problem for him, and he didn't need to wear sweaty ear plugs and muffs. Sometimes, it surprised Janet just how accommodating businesses were, and it wasn't because of welfare—government projects like Affirmative Action or the Americans with Disabilities Act. It was business, the bottom line, and the fact that the disabled were the best fit for many jobs. Society had come a long way from the time when her people stood on corners, hats in hand, begging for food, and money. Some say the label "handicapped" came from those days.

Janet loved the residents of the Center. All of them. Well, most of them. There were two who got on her nerves; a boy and woman she found difficult to like, let alone love. She had to admit, she felt no guilt about her negative feelings for them. We don't live in a perfect world, and there was nothing that required her to love them all. She took people one at a time. Their race, gender, religion, and preferences were not as important as was their individuality. Janet processed people individually. The woman was in her forties and was unpleasantly masculine, bossy, and arrogant. She was also dismissive of Janet. She had the personality traits Janet found herself wanting to avoid. She found herself avoiding the boy, too. Ron frightened her. He was big, reckless, and out of control, and the medications didn't seem to help. Several times he had struck other residents, causing bloody noses and bruised eyes. Each time there was no remorse or promise never again to let frustration turn to violence. To Janet, he was a disaster waiting to happen. He frightened her. The residents had begun to call him "Bad Ron."

Janet went back to her office to make the call to Planned Parenthood. She was one of the few staff members with walls. The others lived and worked in cubicles. She prided herself on the tasteful way she had decorated those walls. The decor included ferns and flowers, not too small or large, a small maple table rather than a cold metal desk, and a wooden filing cabinet. She had only one picture tastefully framed and strategically placed on her table-desk. It was of her, Ben, and their pug, Rosie. It was an action snapshot of their lives rather than a posed, artificial one. It showed them boarding Ben's specially-equipped van and was taken by their neighbor, a retired professor with the photography hobby. Pugs, perhaps the ugliest animals in the kingdom, take great pictures. They are natural showoffs. Ben takes a good one, too. And except for needing to lose ten or fifteen pounds, so did she. For the past five years, Janet knew she was going to lose those excess hip pounds and soon. She even put off buying new outfits knowing that they would be too baggy, what with her new diet and all.

Janet had met Ben in college, and it wasn't love at first sight. She had learned from the past that love at first sight usually required a second look. The man before Ben had been handsome and cocky. It was the cockiness she had found attractive. He was self-assured, convinced of his ability to succeed at anything and everything. They had dated for three years, off and on. About two years into the relationship, Janet had realized he was still looking beyond her for something or someone. She also knew she was still shopping, and he hadn't proven himself worthy. Janet prided herself on her high standards for the mate and father of her yet-to-be-conceived children. She wouldn't settle for just handsome and cocky, there had to be substance. And then she had met Ben.

Janet often thought of Ben during her jogs. Early morning jogs had become yet another arsenal in the battle of the bulge around her hips. Actually, Janet could have been a starved Ethiopian poster child and she still would have jogged early in the mornings. She loved the early morning quiet, crisp air, and the sun rising, bringing a new day of possibilities. She didn't jog far, just two miles around the southern end of the campus and into the small unincorporated township. The campus and city planners had created a wonderful maze of jogging trails with rustic wooden bridges, a tunnel, arrows, bright yellow halogen lights, and yield signs. The path she usually pounded coursed through the campus and along Oak River, where ducks, muskrats, and turtles the size of boulders slipped beneath the muddy Midwestern water. There were the usual early morning joggers, pacing themselves to rapid, deep breathing. Like ships in the night, they would cross paths or overtake each other and nod or simply utter, "Morning." By D-day, July 5th, the day they would leave for Anchorage, Janet hoped to have doubled her distance, endurance, and strength.

As Janet rounded the bend and crossed the first of the three bridges, she pondered Ben and how to break the news. Janet wanted a child. She wanted the intimacy of an infant, the smell of talcum power, dirty diapers, breast feeding, tricycles, and the energy of a toddler. She wanted PTA meetings, Christmas concerts, 8th-grade sock hops, prom dresses, and wedding plans. She wanted to be a mother. Nature was nudging and the time was right. If the past seven years had proven anything, it was that she and Ben could do the family thing. Ben would be a great father, loving yet firm, and he would succeed at hunting and gathering. The Center had a family leave policy that would allow Janet an uninterrupted year to nest. Together, they would create a wonderful home for a lucky boy or girl.

In the past, Ben had been reluctant to talk of children. He managed to change the subject whenever the topic was broached. They had talked of everything and anything, and Ben was characteristically open except about babies and children. A few months ago, Janet had realized that Ben was afraid. Janet knew Ben and admired his tenacity. Fear was not a big part of his life, but she sensed it when the conversation turned to children. Why he was fearful was beyond her comprehension.

Ben is a good man. Oh, Janet realized that was not saying much. Men are men, and Ben, like most of them, didn't have a clue. The good ones are thoughtful, open, caring, committed, and loving. The good ones are easy to laughter. But the good ones think too much like the not-so-good ones. They think it's all about strength, size, power, appearance, and bravado. The good women, Janet knew she was one, were more thoughtful about life, love, and relationships. Her love for Ben had begun in a class they shared in graduate school and gradually blossomed. Each day, their relationship strengthened. He had the little things that are so important. He had the important day-to-day things that made their relationship. Ben is a good man and he doesn't have a clue. Even when they fought, he fought fair, and hurtful remarks were kept to a minimum. When the fighting became too much, he simply got in his van and drove to nowhere in particular. Only once had a fight threatened their existence. Afterward, the emotionally battered combatants had simply returned home and resolved to never let it go too far again. It had frightened them.

Janet's pace picked up as she thought more intently about the important things in life. She entered the brightly lit tunnel that was dug beneath a bicycle path and heard her expensive running shoes slap the track and echo from the red brick walls. Maybe, she thought, Ben wasn't ready. Maybe it was just that he needed time to get comfortable with the idea. For Janet, time was running out. Unlike men, women hear the distant biological clock ticking away uterine opportunities. Janet could hear the clock, and she knew time was running out. Life is timed, like all of the tests she had taken in college. For Janet, the time had come.

Chapter Six

I suppose it is because professors make it look easy. Lecturing looks easy, but it is not. It's demanding, hard work. It can go bad in the blink of an eye. Mine usually go well, but sometimes the clock on the wall crawls on, students appear as decaying zombies, PowerPoint slides or overheads die, and a student with a cold and a honking cough can require more repetitions than usual. Because of my speech disorder, I usually use a microphone, but sometimes it dies too, and there is always the problem of high-pitched feedback. Sometimes, it's all about motivation. You wake up and would just as soon not talk to anyone, let alone a classroom with seventy-five curious minds. Lecturing can also be exhilarating, especially when you're exploring an author famous for his or her insight and wit. It can be the best of times and it can be the worst of them. Lecturing can be a rush.

Janet and I rarely fight or even argue. We did more of it when our relationship was young. I suppose it is because we were staking territory and learning boundaries. I don't know if it is by design or chance, but Janet usually prompts an argument about an hour before my lectures. She announces "Round One" of these emotionally draining events by saying, "We need to talk." This is woman speak for "You're in trouble now." True to form, about an hour before my 2:20 lecture, over ham and cheese sandwiches, she, out of the blue, simply announced that she didn't want to refill her birth control prescription and that "We need to talk." Of course, she caught me in midswallow, and when you have spastic speech muscles, swallowing is also difficult. So, after five attempts to push the mouthful down my dry throat, I was finally able to respond, and it was a pretty pathetic response: "Huh?" What's a guy to say about that type of an announcement? And besides, Janet already knew how this discussion would turn out. She had already planned and predicted the outcome. All she was doing was bringing me up to speed, informing me of this major change in my tenuous life. See, I'm not as dumb as I look.

Right now, I need a pregnant mate like I need another neuromuscular disorder. Hell, let's have a baby and give me multiple sclerosis, too. I'm already off the scale on the stress index. We're not just talking about a baby here. Actually, I'd like a little curtain climber and rug rat brightening up my life. But I know Janet. We're also going to get married. Who'd want to have a child without the benefit of marriage? We're also going to have to get a larger apartment or even our own house. You couldn't raise a child in this one bedroom dump. Of course, "Mother," my soon-to-be mother-in-law, would make a lengthy visit to help with the newborn. Mother has let it be known that Janet could have any man, men without canes and slurred speech. Mother has let it be known that with me, Janet was bringing her work home. Mother believes Janet lives with me only out of pity. Mother can't seem to have an unexpressed thought! Add to these stressors the fact that I'm up for tenure, and either it will be granted or I will be given a terminal contract. I'll either have a job for life or be unemployed. Announcing that she didn't want to fill a prescription is a pretty mean thing to do, especially an hour before my lecture. Too bad the Americans with Disabilities Act didn't cover this.

So after this bomb was dropped in my lap, so to speak, I managed to get to the lecture hall. Plop-slide, plop-slide, plop-slide. Today, there were no grateful librarians or children to rescue from terrorists. My burden was too great. What if I were denied tenure, terminated, and penniless, with an expensive, mother-in-law filled apartment and a new mouth to feed? Maybe now is not the right time. It's not that I'm not a pessimist, it's just that I'm a realist. Maybe now is not the right time.

With my mind as far from Chaucer as England is from the United States, I tried to teach about metaphors, similes, and personification. Lecturing is different for a gimp professor than for one with normal limbs and speech. A normal professor can wander his or her ideas, misspeak, and lose trains of thought. It happens to normal professors all of the time. But when you have crutches and distorted speech, those normal byproducts of thought can cause rumors of mental incompetence, which obviously goes hand-in-hand with cerebral palsy. Students begin wondering if the good professor has bad thinking. Impaired thinking is a death blow for professors. Students don't like paying tuition to hear the rambling of the retarded or demented. So, I tried hard to keep my mind on the subject at hand, periodically reviewing my woes in my mind. I finally got into a rhythm and managed to stimulate a lively, if not irrelevant, discussion.

One student with a bright tattoo on his shoulder of an American flag surrounding a Saturday night special was taking issue with another student's comment about the Bible and personification. She was one of the new breed of students I have seen gracing the campus during the past few years. I call them Bohemians, and the only thing lacking is Paris of the 1930s, the Left Bank of La Seine, and Hemingway. They hang around coffee shops, smoke cigarettes, and wear berets. They rage against the machine. She remarked that religion personifies the universe, gives humanness, and even worse, maleness, to things not human. God is a man, he had a son, there is communication in the form of prayer, yada, yada, yada. She certainly caught the essence of personification but also the ire of the Christians in the class. I let them argue and debate as I silently pondered responsibilities and my frail shoulders to support them. Finally, the hand of the clock crept to dismissal time, and I was able to bring an end to the class. As I plop-slid toward the door, the Bohemian approached me. She muttered something about how I should be more directive in class and keep the narrow-minded from wasting time of the good minds. She said she felt uncomfortable in my class.

"Why are the broad-minded suddenly so narrow-minded about my time management?" Realizing I had actually said that aloud to the Bohemian, I immediately began to qualify the unintended remark. The Bohemian looked startled at first but picked up the verbal gauntlet. She said something about feeling intimidated and began to whine that the faithful Christians' ideas distressed her good senses. She started down the victim road, professing how life, daddy, and society had done her wrong, wailing on and on about injustices, capitalism, and oppression. My back began to hurt. I can't stand too long in one place without getting these sharp pains in my back. I looked around for a place to sit. It appeared that this one-sided discussion was going to continue.

We were alone in the aisle of the classroom. I realized that I had never really looked at her, and until now, she was just another beret-wearing face in the class. She was in her early twenties and actually quite attractive. She had full lips, reddish-brown hair, and eyes tinted by greenish contact lenses. She dressed in black. She also had a superior, self-righteous air about her. The Bohemian's speech was punctuated with all of the politically correct buzz words. I listened intently to her, not because I wanted to, but because I couldn't get a word in edgewise. I tried to defend my time management, but she interrupted and corrected me. Apparently, I have a lot to learn about the evils of the world. And then it came out of my untenured mouth. It simply sprang from my mouth, and I was helpless to stop it. I said she had a constipation problem and she appeared bloated. Oh, heck, I actually said she was full of shit. My back was hurting, Janet's prescription was on my mind, my crutches were cutting into my wrists, and I was blocked from escaping her talk-show diatribe. It just came out. Well, that energized her. She promptly notified me that my time-management, oppression, and callousness would be reported to the Dean and several of the hordes of committees established to protect her from being uncomfortable. She let me know that she had been empowered since Head Start and that I'd pay for "dissen" her. Then, finally, she stormed out of the classroom and I felt relief. Had I known that was all I needed to say to rid her from my life, I would have said it sooner. I felt like shouting that the toilet was down the hall and to the right. Whew.

As I plop-slide back to my office, I realized that I had created yet another problem to add to the mounting list. Now, I would have to deal with radical feminists and other hate groups set on ridding the world of evil. Committees of sensitive, Alan Alda-type liberal professors would review my callousness and tisk, tisk their disdain. My views on the world would be explored and examined in excruciating detail. Oh, some of them would excuse my behavior because I am disabled. There are those on campus who embrace racism, sexism, and harassment when it is done by the right people for the good of us all. This would be awful. I'll probably be sent to a Cambodian re-education camp to learn sensitivity. The prize of tenure would certainly be denied. This all because of my big, spastic mouth.

Chapter Seven

My leg hurt and I do mean hurt. And I was cold. The Cessna in the stream was barely recognizable. I had the ironic thought that with two more payments, the crumpled mess would be all mine. But we were alive, more or less, and I had to think about getting us home and medical care. Oh God, the pain in my leg was unbearable, and I was losing blood. I got sick to my stomach when I saw the white bone protruding from above my knee. I started to get light-headed. I saw the four of them and realized that we may not have survived the crash after all. Four retards, miles from help, stranded in the outback of Alaska. My only consolation was that I did my best and that comforted me. I passed out from the pain.

Trevor carried Nicole to a grassy clearing where sunlight cast long shadows. He laid her down gently on the pine needles serving as a mat. She was crying, wet, and cold, but she was alive. Trevor was shivering both from fear and the cold. Trevor's left hand had a puncture wound, but it had stopped bleeding. Elroy had a nasty cut on his back and shoulder, and the blood had stained his wet shirt a pinkish hue. He also felt his right side and knew something was broken. It hurt when he breathed. Rusty was standing next to a large boulder looking at the bright yellow airplane occasionally rolling and sliding down the stream, uttering: "Mayde," "Mayde," Mayde."

Four souls with a combined IQ under 300 looked at where fate had deposited them. From the vantage point of the nearby pine trees, they sat, either crying or quiet, with Elroy shaking the shoulder of the unconscious pilot, saying: "Wake-up, Mr. Pilot," "Wake-up, please." Nicole sobbed as Trevor, kneeling next to her, held her hand, and tried to process the frightening events. Rusty was now using his fingers to strobe the sunlight, barely detectable over the surrounding mountains, and he began to rock back and forth.

From the canyon ridge above the Dolores River, five humans sit or lay quietly while the yellow wreckage of the airplane bobs and slides in the roaring, picturesque river. From the top of the mountains paralleling the canyon, only several blurry dots are visible, nothing really distinguishing them from the surroundings. From the distant view of a commercial airliner shooting across the Alaskan sky and trailing white, dissipating vapor, nothing of the crashed flying machine or frightened souls could be seen. And from the global view of communication satellites, where the long Alaskan and Canadian coast line stretched for thousands of miles, islands and glaciers could be distinguished, but there was nothing to signal the plight of the five survivors, nothing but rugged wilderness, wild hungry animals, and the life and death drama that was to unfold.

Chapter Eight

Janet knew things were not going well between Ben and her. It had been weeks since their busy schedules had allowed any form of intimacy. She hoped it was their busy schedules, but in the back of her mind, she feared that he was avoiding her sexually. Each night, he was either already asleep when she came to bed or he stayed up late to read papers, often sleeping on the old green and brown couch until daybreak. She knew he was troubled about work. He had told her of some verbal altercation with one of his students. As she increased her jogging pace, she began to wonder where all of these stressors were going to take them. She was feeling out of control. It worried her.

It was unusually warm and she was already sweating. Birds were chirping, and in the distance you could hear the early risers speeding down State Street. She could feel her heart pounding in her chest, her hair bouncing, and a tightness in her knees. It wasn't pain, just tightness, and she put more spring in her run. Jogging has so many benefits. It is healing to the mind and soul, a form of meditation. It opens pores and blood vessels. The lungs breathe deeply and the heart grows stronger. Leg and hip muscles strengthen and become firm. The morning jogger greets the day robustly and with energy. But jogging jars the hips and knees. It takes a toll on joints, but it is a small price to pay. Janet was committed to jogging. She knew she would eventually be one of those little old ladies jogging, walking really, early in the mornings in some retirement community in the South. Jogging was a permanent part of her life. She wished Ben could share the joys of jogging with her.

When she returned to their apartment, Ben had already gone to work. What possible business did he have at the University at 7:30 A.M.? He had made the coffee and left the newspaper carefully folded at her end of the table. Janet showered, dried her hair, and as she closed the door to their apartment, she realized that it had become far too quiet. Janet and Ben had begun to co-exist.

It came out of the blue. There was no warning, no indication before Ron struck her hard in the face, knocking her to the ground. Janet had been teaching him the finer points of sorting recyclable paper, how colored paper went in the blue drum and all others in the yellow one, when it happened. They were alone and in the large, brightly lit supply room, the door partially open. It never occurred to Janet that Ron would strike her, let alone drop to his knees, place his hands around her throat, and try to choke the life from her. But he was determined to kill. With her strong running legs, she kicked at his groin, but her foot missed the sensitive target. She tried to turn on her stomach and then knock him backward, but he was too strong and too determined. She tried to scream, but his hands stopped the flow of air carrying the cry for help. In the corner of her eyes, she saw Rusty peeking through the partially opened door. He was staring at the violence, captivated by it. He was too frightened and confused to help. She knew he would be a nonverbal witness to her murder. She kept fighting and struggling, and then she began to weaken.

Elroy usually never let Janet out of his sight when she was at the Center. But he and a supervisor had driven the Center's truck to a grocery store to pick up donated bread, buns, cookies, and cakes for the Day Old store. Day old? Yeah, right. Even the residents at the Center knew that foodstuffs in the store were older than a day. Elroy loved that part of his job at the Center. He got to ride in the big truck, high above the other traffic. He always purchased a soda from the grocery store after the work of loading was done. On the ride back to the Center, he'd also bum a smoke from the driver and was just learning how to inhale without coughing. He knew he was the envy of everyone watching him riding shotgun in that large truck. Ah, it was a wonderful life. He loved trips to the grocery stores.

As the truck backed into the loading dock with the beep, beep, beep warning all to run for cover, Elroy looked around for Janet. He knew she would be lonesome for him, sad and dreaming of his return. She had probably spent the past hour searching the Center for him. But she was nowhere to be found. After the truck had stopped and the engine turned off, Elroy began searching for her. As he walked by a door, he saw Rusty with his back to the wall, strobing, and muttering: "Dodear, Dodear." Elroy thought that was strange even for Rusty.

When he opened the door, he couldn't believe his eyes. Bad Ron was hurting Janet. All of Elroy's life, he had been taught never to be violent, never to strike or hurt anyone—never. And Elroy fostered ill will toward no one. He loved people, all of them, even Bad Ron. What to do? He went over to two struggling bodies and shouted, "Stop it, stop it, please." Oh, what to do? "Stop it, now." He began to dance around them, his mind blocked. Then, Elroy reached down and grabbed Bad Ron by his jacket and threw him through the air and into the wall. Slowly, Janet's screams became louder, and finally staff and supervisors came to her rescue. Elroy began to cry.

Chapter Nine

I usually eat lunch at home. One of the perks of professoring is that you can come and go as you wish, as long as you keep regular office hours and, of course, teach your classes. But today the Chair of the Department wanted to talk to me. We decided to have lunch at one of the small restaurants in the International Center. The International Center is the hub of the campus and sits next to the library complex, in full view of Bell Tower. The Bell Tower announces the hour and half-hour with clarion music and is the beating heart of the campus. It is a splendid addition to this beautiful campus and is surrounded by rolling hills, ancient weeping willow trees, and a concert area created out of grass, bushes, and flowers. It's just below the campus stadium, which seats nearly a hundred thousand football fans. On Football Saturdays, you can hear the roar of the crowd for miles. I've had season passes since I was a student.

Bob Charles is a fine person, for a guy with two first names. He's been Chair of the Department for twelve years. Twelve years is a lifetime in administration. He's seen it all come and go over the years. Every issue has been dealt with, every contingency planned, every conflict addressed. University politics are really cutthroat. I suppose it's because you have intelligent and educated people with a sense of self-importance. But, I swear, I've seen more maturity at the Center. Once during the dreaded weekly faculty meeting, a faculty member almost threw herself on the floor kicking and wailing because she didn't get her way. Another fellow actually stood up and stormed out of the room while hurling epitaphs at us. These were over course scheduling conflicts. The faculty meetings are held in the department conference room, or the "viper pit" as one assistant professor now calls it.

Bob was uncharacteristically late so I decided to get something to eat. I have a class in about an hour. At this cafe, you must pass through a line, plopping food on a tray that you slide along four stainless steel bars. I suppose that is a convenience for most people, but for me, with two metal canes protruding from my arms, it's problematic. But I was hungry, time was short, and there were no options. So, I plop-slide to the cashier and told her of my predicament. Actually, I told her twice. I have to remember to open my mouth widely and say each sound as clearly as possible or my punishment will be "Pardon? You need kelp with that ocean spray?" She was a tiny person but well-proportioned, and I liked her matter-of-fact manner. She asked me what I wanted and where I was sitting. I paid for the food in advance, and when there was a lull in the action, she brought the tray to me. I smiled and said, "Thank you."

"I'm sorry I'm late," Bob Charles said as he arrived. "I would have been here sooner but I didn't leave early enough." Bob has that droll English humor I find confusing. I never know when to laugh or even if I should. I told him it was no problem and that I started lunch without him. Ever polite, he excused himself, walked to the stack of trays and began to select the most bland of food. I had heard through the grapevine that he had something irritable residing in his digestive tract and could appease it only with soft, tasteless food.

Bob took a seat next to me, a little too close for my sexual comfort. Apparently, our conversation was to be private and intimate. He had his usual worried look on his face. He was dressed in his typical administrative uniform: blue suit, red tie, and spit-shined wingtip shoes. Bob has the kind of body not designed for suit-wearing. Every suit he owns fits poorly, like clothing on a monkey. They fit too tightly in some places and too loosely in others. Bob should wear greasy coveralls like the ones worn by mechanics. The coveralls could have his name sown on them: Bob Charles, Chair. He'd finally look comfortable.

Pity is the worst. It is by far the worst part of being disabled, and Bob occasionally teeters over the line separating it from compassion. I don't want no stinking pity. Pity belittles me while providing an ego boost for the ones doing it. Fortunately, I knew Bob's purpose when he teetered toward pity. It was to help me and to make my life a little easier. Bob was as close to a friend as I had in the Department. As he began to eat the nonirritating sandwich and slurp his bland soup, he announced, "You're in trouble with the Promotion and Tenure Committee." Between bites, he explained that my student evaluations, while good, were not in the upper quartile for the department, and several students said I was hard to understand. And although I had published two novels, several articles in literary journals, and one in a national weekly magazine, the quality of my scholarship was "borderline." "Publish or perish," he said. Adding to the litany of bad news, he said I was also being investigated for the heinous crime of insensitivity. Apparently, the Bohemian had followed through on her threat. Bob put his hand on my shoulder and said, "We'll get through this. You know you have my support, but it'll be a battle." And then Bob made me angry. In so many roundabout words, he said I should play the "disabled card." I should use it as a preemptive strike. I should go to one of the committees charged with making college comfortable and say that I was being bullied *because of my disabilities.* I should become the victim. Once again, my spastic mouth took over, and I reactively told him, "Sure, Bob, I'll also buy a beret, take up smoking, and start wearing black." He didn't have a clue what that meant, and I didn't feel the need to explain. I was angry.

I have had conflicts with several of the Promotion and Tenure Committee members. One member, a woman who reminded me of "Mother," had complained that I teach too much white, European male literature. Other committee members were simply jealous of my novels. Two had commented that I pandered to the pathetic populace. They condemned the books because the great unwashed masses actually bought and read them. One of the comments on my peer review said I lacked "collegiality." That's professor-speak for not being right-minded. People expect me to be ever so politically correct, liberal on politics, antiguns, antismoking, anti this, that, and the other thing, and vocal for massive government programs to rescue the downtrodden. I'm not, never have been, never will be, and it upsets people. Too bad. Deal with it. Oh, the viper pit was active during my tenure deliberations.

Bob was right. I was in trouble with the Committee, but it wasn't because of my cerebral palsy, slurred speech, raspy voice, and gimpness. It was because they disapproved of my performance. They simply disliked me for being me. You gotta love people like that. I was disliked and disapproved of for all of the right reasons, the same ones that had caused three professors in the past year to be denied promotion and tenure. It was the same petty crap, and I admired them for it. No way would I play the disabled card. Let the cards fall where they may. Some things are more important than promotion and tenure. Some things are more important than job security. Some things are more important than happiness.

About the time I finished explaining to Bob my reasons for not playing the disabled card, my cell phone rang. It was a social worker at the hospital telling me that Janet had been admitted. She quickly told me that Janet was in good condition and that she was just being held for observation. When my heart stopped racing and my hands shaking, I told Bob of the family emergency and went to the hospital. I met the social worker in the lobby and together we went to Janet's room. I couldn't believe my eyes.

Janet was asleep. A nurse said she had been sedated. She lay between the crisp, white hospital sheets with her long, dark hair flowing over a small pillow. Sleeping Beauty with a huge black, red, and blue eye. There were stitches running from her eyebrow. When I saw the bluish finger marks around her long, sensual neck, I got sick to my stomach and felt the need to go to the bathroom. For an instant, I thought I'd caught something irritable from Bob. I felt tears run down my eyes, and I went to the window and looked at the busy parking lot. Oddly, I felt both joy and rage. I wanted to hug Janet, tell her I loved her, and then drive to the Center and kill Bad Ron.

Janet never talked about it, to me anyway. After she was discharged from the hospital, I took her home and did my best to nurse her psychologically and physically. I catered to her every need. She read and did needlepoint. She slept late into the mornings, which was unusual. For two weeks, she cleaned the apartment, polished our sparse silverware, talked on the phone to "Mother," and did laundry. She asked about my work, cared for me, and kept busy. Every time I broached the subject, thinking it would be good for her to talk about it, she politely refused to relive it. On the Sunday morning before she returned to work, while we ate bagels in bed and read the *Sunday Journal,* I again tried to get her to talk about it. No way. I realized that for Janet, the subject was closed. Some things are too private, too personal, and we would never discuss it. If that was how she was going to deal with her attempted murder, then so be it. Whatever it takes. Monday morning, Janet woke early, dawned her jogging clothes, and resumed her life. Bad Ron was history. I did note that around her neck hung a small silver whistle and a gray tube of extra-strength pepper spray. That afternoon, I went to Big Jake's Guns and Liquor and signed a document promising that I wasn't insane or criminal. I bought a .22 caliber semiautomatic pistol and placed it in the small drawer next to my side of the bed. For Janet, Bad Ron may be history, but he had taken my security and the gun helped restore it. $395.00 is a small price to pay for a sense of security.

Chapter Ten

Finals week drew a bad semester to a close. Faculty are required to attend every other graduation ceremony, but I attend them all. I love the pomp and circumstance, the marching, the gowns, and the elated students with conferred degrees. I listen to the speakers talk of lofty goals and sadly note the end of an important part of life. Caps are thrown in the air, students and parents cry, and faculty are hugged. It is a time of beginnings and endings. For me, I feared it was more ending than beginning. The Promotion and Tenure Committee had sent their secretive report to the Dean and Provost. I would be notified of their decision after our return from Alaska. Apparently, there was some delay with my application. I hate the waiting. I was getting a little edgy.

I was avoiding the issue of children and unfilled prescriptions like the plague. Maybe the time wasn't right for another mouth to feed. For three weeks, Janet and I simply caught glimpses of each other going through doors, driving out of the apartment complex, eating sandwiches, and falling to sleep. For the first week after Janet returned to work, sex was out of the question. I knew the daily birth control pills had run out and danger lurked in the bedroom. I could rid sex from my life. Monks, priests, and nerds did it all of the time. No man ever died from a lack of sex. I can do celibacy standing on my head.

I breezed through the first week. During the second week, I continued to avoid Janet and bed, though I did find myself watching her walk and talk with more interest. She has soft hands. The nape of her neck is as sensual as her smell. I love the curve of her body as she lies on the couch, particularly where waist meets hip. Janet also wears reading glasses; need I say more? One morning, I found myself studying newspaper ads for bras and panties. Those models were certainly shameless. I recalled from my youth nasty pictures in *Playboy* of wanton women wearing about the same amount of clothing as seen in those ads that today boldly take up an entire page of a newspaper.

At work, I found it difficult to maintain eye-contact with busty women. By the third week, a millennium without sex, I began rethinking my position on children. Like I said, I was getting a little edgy. So, like a remorseful puppy, one night I left the stack of term papers, slipped into bed with Janet, and began caressing her, my pathetic nonverbal way of initiating. She met me with open, unprotected arms. What the heck, maybe the time was right for children. Let's cross that bridge later. Afterward, I felt pretty good about my resolve. Three weeks of sexual self-denial. Not bad. Janet slept smugly, all along knowing how this would work out. I slept an entire night for the first time in three weeks. I woke the next morning refreshed and renewed, but knowing one thing for certain: I am a weak man. Like my cerebral palsy, it's just another part of my life to accept. I took solace in the fact that most men are sexual cripples.

The night before we were to leave for Anchorage, the Center was abuzz with excitement. Rusty was constantly strobing, rocking, and uttering "cheska," a reference to something no one could decipher. We had given him a map with yellow markings showing our path from Anchorage to Fairbanks and then to the wilderness cabin. He kept pointing to it and saying, "cheska." Elroy wanted to share a suitcase with Janet and trailed her from room to room. He always managed to be standing between me and Janet, with his back to me. He's a cocky one, all right. Anastasia locked herself in her bedroom, and we had to get a master key to console her. Nicole and Trevor packed together, talking about necessary items. Janet had to remove half of what they packed and replace it with items a little more practical for an Alaskan adventure. For some reason, Trevor believed shoe polish and a small reading lamp would be necessary. I could almost understand the shoe polish, but reading was not one of Trevor's strengths. Nicole carefully placed her birth control pills in the small carrying case full of toiletries. Janet and Melissa had taught her the intricacies of planned parenthood. Tomorrow at 6:50 A.M. we would begin our great adventure. Late that evening Janet and I returned home, and once again, I set my swimmers free to find her elusive egg. I was beginning to like the idea of being a father. I was a lot more relaxed.

I had met with the "Committee" charged with reviewing my conduct with the Bohemian, and it wasn't as awful as I thought it would be. I expected a committee of spineless wonders, strapped to their chairs so they wouldn't tumble to the floor. But they patiently listened to the Bohemian and then gave me my turn. She went on and on about her comfort level and how I had probably ruined her life, a job began by her daddy and our founding fathers. The pain she felt was incredible. When it was my turn, I simply held my ground. There would be no remorse and no undoing. As far as I was concerned, I had a God-given right to say anything and everything I felt was important. Notice that I said God-given right. You see, I don't have much physical freedom, what with canes and spastic muscles. Consequently, freedom of speech is very important to me. I don't believe the government, or anyone else for that matter, has the right to control someone's speech. Period, and it's not open for discussion. How's that for a contradiction? Freedom of speech is too important to me, society, evolution, and life. And a lot of soldiers have died face down in the mud to protect it. I'll say what's on my mind and if the powers that be don't like it, too bad. Arrest me, fire me, execute me. I'll say what's on my mind and damn the consequences. I'll also run my courses the way I see fit. I believe in academic freedom. As I told the "Committee," let the Bohemian get several degrees, teach for nearly a decade, age for two more, and then I might be interested in her myopic opinions of my course management. I told the "Committee" of her constipation and bloating problem.

I was surprised that many on the committee shared my views. Oh, there were several who talked of limits of freedom. I let them talk and even listened, though I've heard it before. I didn't feel unbearable discomfort at what they had to say, even though I couldn't have disagreed more. Finally, the committee reached a decision that there would be no censure or reprimand. One member commented to the Bohemian that if other people's ideas made her so uncomfortable, maybe she was not ready for college; maybe she needed a little time off for introspection. At the conclusion of the meeting, I felt elated. The Bohemian stormed from the Faculty Senate Hearing Room convinced of yet more oppression, and I knew she would continue to rage against the machine. Life goes on. In my office later that evening, I sent an e-mail to the Bohemian. I apologized for my insensitivity.

Chapter Eleven

Someone had wrapped my leg with a tattered shirt. The pain had now diminished to a constant throb accompanied by a burning sensation. I was still light-headed but alive. I knew that below the blood-soaked tattered shirt, the bone of my leg was still protruding from the skin. Curiously, I thought of how the makeshift bandage would protect my body from invasion by ants and bloodsucking maggots. My life-savior was shaking my shoulder, demanding that I awaken. I pushed his hand aside, and slowly, painfully, slid myself into a half-sitting position with my back to a boulder. He stopped talking and awaited my leadership. I realized that unless my distress call was heard by other pilots, my instructions were going to be simple: "Prepare to kiss your butts goodbye."

The sun was setting. Well, at this time of year in Alaska, it really doesn't set. It just gets lower in the sky. But it was dark because of the trees, canyon, and mountains. I was cold and I knew we needed a fire. A fire would provide warmth and also a beacon for search planes. I told my savior to get kindling and wood together, and I would somehow muster the strength to use my lighter to get a fire started. He and the one called "Trevor" quickly rose to the occasion and soon had enough down and dead wood for a warming beacon. Dead grass and moss crumpled under the kindling soon burst into flame, and fire was released. Another irony. I was happy that my attempts to quit smoking were unsuccessful and put the prized lighter back in my pocket. I told the passengers to keep the fire burning. I said it loudly and several times. They're retarded after all. Again, I passed out.

Rusty, Nicole, Trevor, and Elroy moved close to the small fire. It warmed them physically and psychologically. Soon, everyone had fallen asleep, not so much from fatigue but as a temporary escape from the fear. The crackling of the fire and deep breathing were drowned in the roar of the Dolores River. Soon, the fire died as the passengers slept. Hours later, Elroy awoke. He again shook the shoulder of the pilot. But, there was no response. He looked around. Nicole and Trevor slept in each other's arms. Rusty was awake, but he just stared at the smoke rising from the dead fire. Elroy thought of Janet and knew she must be worried about him. He was cold and his side felt like a spear had penetrated it. Elroy knew he must find her. Forgetting the "Hug a Tree" lecture, he stood up, left the camp, and began the search for Janet and the rescue party he knew she would be leading. Rusty continued to stare at the smoke rising from the dead fire. Nicole, without opening her eyes, pulled Trevor closer, and they shared lifesaving body heat.

Nyle was from Liverpool but had lived and worked in Alaska for twenty-four years. His only regret was that in Alaska women are rare. It's about five to one in most towns and cities, and in real Alaska, the vast wilderness, it was more like a hundred to one for unattached females. After a quarter of a century, he was still searching for the woman to share his life. But Nyle was already in love. His first and only love was flying, and being a bush pilot in Alaska was a dream come true. Each day was a scenic adventure. Today, he was taking a young couple to Tucktoyuktuk for a hiking and camping honeymoon when he heard the "May Day." He was short on fuel and knew an immediate response was dangerous. Two downed planes would help no one. He contacted Fairbanks Tower and told them of the emergency. They had heard part of the distress call but were unable to detect anything on radar. Air Search and Rescue was alerted, and pilots from Fairbanks and surrounding areas left jobs and family to search for one of their kind.

Chapter Twelve

If you are a people watcher, like me, airports are voyeur heaven; thousands of people rushing, waiting, drinking, eating, and shuffling heavy luggage down wide corridors. After the Center's bus deposited us at the loading zone, where bright red signs threatened to execute us if, even for a second, there was loitering, we became part of the human mass swelling to gates and airplanes. After our luggage was placed on conveyer belts and sped off to parts unknown, we began the long journey to Gate 17 in Terminal 3.

I don't know whether normal people are stared at during these journeys, but we were the objects of people's attention. Now I know how famous rock groups feel when they embark and debark airplanes. I suppose we did look a sight. Janet, lead singer and female sex object, took the lead and set the pace, followed by Drummer Rusty strobing and occasionally uttering "cheska." I brought up the rear, following the rhythm section, Anastasia, Trevor, and Nicole. Our pace was slow, but we had plenty of time. If normals must be at the airport two hours before takeoff, we knew to double the lead time. We politely refused the offer to ride on one of the golf carts and be rushed to the gate. That seemed like cheating. Let our great adventure begin in this airport and the lesson of independence and character start with the long hike to the first of three airplanes. As we made our way most people stared, but they kept going. Some actually stopped just to observe us. Two children shouted, "Look Daddy." Twice, I stopped and returned their stares and once, just for the fun of it, I strobed like Rusty.

Over the years, I have learned that airport travelers are not being rude or mean at their unbroken eye-contact. It's unconscious on their part. They just see something unusual, and it takes time for them to process it. They're like Trevor. It takes time to figure out what the heck is going on. They wonder about our destination, purpose, and means. They wonder who is retarded and who is in charge. On a deeper level, they ponder the meaning of life. Why are we the way we are, and they spared our plight? Oh, some are distressed that we exist and are angry that we don't know our place. Aren't there institutions for our kind? Doesn't government have places where we are cared for by well-spent tax dollars? Twice, I have heard drunks at airports make unkind jokes. Of course, they're crippled by alcohol, a fear of flying, and a tendency to shout their nonsense.

I watch them, too. I see families off to reunions, divorced dads sending children back to their biological mothers, grandparents heading to winter retreats, and students returning to their studies. There are the business travelers with plans of hostile takeovers. The most interesting of travelers are the lovers rejoicing or despairing. They hug and share long kisses. They stroke arms and backs waiting for the painful separation. They squeal and embrace with smiles so permanent they will need to be surgically removed. It is a drama watching people at airports, and we appeared to be the main act. I plop-slide onto one of the people movers, you know, those conveyor belts for people. My canes leave far more quickly than my reluctant feet, and for an instant, I'm stretched like an elastic band. Trevor and Nicole appear to enjoy the people mover the most. It's like a ride at Disneyland but without the long lines. They share puppy dog looks of intimacies and secrets only young lovers know. There is a glow about them.

We finally reach the gate and begin the long wait before we can speed through the thin atmosphere. Hurry up and wait. I stack my canes on the next plastic seat and continue the theater. Just who would be sharing the first leg of our adventure with us? It seems there will be the usual compositions: old, young, colored, uncolored, tall, short, loud, quiet, business, and recreational. It will be a diverse group of sardines in the tin. I take comfort in seeing the babies and toddlers. I know that God and pilots would never let the plane crash with such precious cargo. Oh oh, Nicole and Trevor are holding hands and looking deeply into each other eyes as they talk of their world. I'm envious at the magic they share, but I look to see if there are ugly people on our adventure. Young love among the physically and mentally disabled sometimes brings out the worst in people. But, if facial expressions show what people are thinking, then our compatriots on this journey are not distressed. We are with the live and let live crowd.

Finally, the attendant announces that those passengers crippled by success, spastic muscles, and small children can board first. Ordinarily, I board with the rest of the sardines, refusing to play the disabled card. But, because of my companions, this time I play the game. As I give my boarding pass to the uniformed attendant, he announces that our party will experience "First Class." Apparently, on this flight there was a shortage of the rich, and the airline, knowing our defects, bumped us to the elite. We would have more room for crutches, seizures, strobing, drooling, and to be able stretch out on the long flight to Anchorage. We would also have hot facial towels (I make a mental note to see how Rusty handles hot towels), unlimited beverages, and attention. We would have two choices of meals and all the peanuts that can be digested. We boarded first and were the envy of all others shuffling down the aisle to their second-class status.

The flight to Anchorage was long and unremarkable. I was able to sit by Janet only after convincing Elroy that the audio headset worked best in a window seat. The airplane was one of the jumbo jets, a DC something or other. We were pampered by the flight attendant and watched an old Disney movie about dogs and cats trying to return home. Rusty strobed and rocked during the entire flight, much to the irritation of the passenger sitting behind him. Anastasia slept some of the flight or simply reclined in her seat with her eyes closed. Twice she took Rusty's strobing hand and forced it in his lap. Rusty was also getting on Anastasia's nerves. Nicole and Trevor sat together in the seats closest to the curtain separating us from the second-class riffraff. I don't think they stopped holding hands even during the meal. The flight was smooth and comfortable. Most of the time, the clouds below us blocked the view. I read, slept, and ate enough peanuts to fill a small elephant. Janet spent more time in the restroom than all of us. Flying makes her airsick.

Across the aisle was another first classer sitting next to her husband. She was one of those direct people who simply asked about us. She was curious. I told her of the Center and the grant. She asked very intelligent questions about Rusty, Anastasia, and me. We struck up an easy, temporary friendship. I wondered if the quality of conversation was as good in second class.

Chapter Thirteen

Nyle made a perfect three-point landing. The Piper Cub, a tail-dragger, touched down lightly and simultaneously on all three wheels. Soon, a large truck with two grades of fuel paralleled his airplane. Within twenty minutes, the Piper's wing tanks were full. Nyle grabbed a sandwich and coffee from the vending machine, went to the bathroom, and was in the cockpit in time to sign for the fuel. He decided to forego the preflight check, got tower clearance, and soon was racing to the Dolores River. The nighttime sun, dim and barely perceptible over the horizon, provided enough light for six hours of searching. He decided to drop below the canyon and simply follow the Dolores River to the inlet. Flying low and fast through a canyon was dangerous, but the sense of speed was exhilarating. Only good pilots dared do it, and Nyle was a good pilot. At 120 knots he sped through the Dolores Canyon, the roar of the propeller and engine frightening several fishing grizzlies. They ran in search of safety from the huge bird of prey. He hoped he wouldn't meet some other search plane coming the opposite direction.

I awoke again, my leg throbbing and my head pounding with pain. I saw that the fire had died. I shouted for Elroy and Trevor. Trevor came to me, but there was

no sign of Elroy. I asked Trevor where Elroy was, and after a brief delay, he said:
"Janet. He find Janet." My stomach turned to a knot, and I knew that there would be
the report of at least one fatality. Damn it. I thought of sending Trevor to find him,
but I knew he would also get lost, and that would lead to two reports of fatalities. I
shouted for Elroy to return to the safety of the camp, but there was no response. The
Dolores River was too loud and I was too weak. With Trevor's help, we again
achieved fire. I hoped Elroy was not too far away to see the smoke. I wondered if he
would have the brains to return to camp. I slipped into unconsciousness, certain that
their frightened faces would be my last image of this world.

After thirty minutes of walking, Elroy was hopelessly lost. He could see
nothing familiar, and even the sound of the river was gone. He was frightened and cold. Elroy could think of nothing but Janet as he began to run in
the direction he knew would lead to their reunion. He ran for nearly an hour
through trees and bushes before he collapsed on a big smooth rock. He
started to cry. Then, in the distance, he heard a low-pitched growl. Frightened at the sound of what he knew was a hungry bear the size of a truck,
Elroy again ran. He ran and ran and ran. Finally, he sat with his back to a
large pine tree.

About an hour from Tucktoyucktuk, Nyle saw smoke spiraling from
the canyon. Knowing that slow, low, and heavy was dangerous for any airplane, he climbed above the canyon and circled it. He made three low but fast
passes over the source of the smoke. Each time he saw the yellow wreckage
of the airplane and several people. He continued to circle above the crash site
while he radioed Fairbanks. A search and rescue helicopter was diverted to
his location and soon was setting down at a small clearing just above a bend
in the river. He saw the rescuers rush to the downed airplane and the frightened passengers. They waved and announced that they had the rescue under
control. Nyle then pushed the throttle forward on his Piper and began a gradual upward spiral to clear the high canyon walls. He dipped wings several
time in farewell and began the flight home. On the forest floor, Elroy looked
up, wiped his tears, and saw the airplane shoot across the sky.

Chapter Fourteen

Janet had thrown up three mornings in a row. Locked in the small restroom
of the airplane, she tried to kneel in such a way as to contain it. The good
news was that there was nothing to empty from her stomach. The better news
was that she was pregnant. The bad news was that she was pregnant *now*. As
she flushed the vacuum-driven toilet, she thought that perhaps Ben was
right. Maybe now was not the right time. Janet had miscalculated. Apparently, it is a lot easier to get pregnant than she had thought. After reaching
her seat, Janet watched Anchorage approach through the small portal. She
was surprised at how large the city was.

The huge jet, a "heavy" as it is called by the tower, touched down as smooth and gentle as a seagull. Janet helped the adventurers disembark. After collecting themselves, they walked and shuffled to a small cafe. They feasted on very expensive sandwiches, slices of pizza, hamburgers, and colas. Watching them eat, Janet thought how fortunate she was to be able to share this time with them. So many people in the world are unremarkable. They strive to wear the same clothes, express the same sentiments, and live ordinary, mundane lives. In the world of people, most are like bland vanilla ice cream in a store offering thirty-one flavors. But not her people. They entered this world different and unique. Her people viewed and responded to it on their own terms and in their own exceptional ways. They had innocence uncontaminated by mediocrity.

Rusty sat on the edge of his chair chewing mouthful after mouthful of potato salad. He was completely caught up in the sight, texture, smell, and taste of it. Janet could tell that for Rusty, nothing else in the world existed but the yellow food; his world *was* potato salad. Anastasia was picking at her pizza slice. She had carefully removed the pastrami, olives, peppers, and chunks of sausage. Between bites, she cautiously scanned the dinning room looking for threats and danger. Her mother's drinking problem had caused Anastasia to be fearful of strangers. Janet chuckled silently to herself as she saw Nicole and Trevor arguing about napkins and straws. Apparently, someone neglected to place them on their tray. Were clouds brewing in paradise? Would too much closeness cause a spat? Elroy sat next to Janet eating nearly $20.00 worth of airport food. Janet had to remind him to slow down. He had a tendency to gulp an entire meal. Janet lacked elbow room because, as usual, Elroy sat too close to her. And then there was Ben, the father of her unborn child. He sat quietly, slowly picking at a hamburger and fries, lost in thought.

Boarding the smaller jet was quick and easy, even though they had to suffer the indignities of second class. It was a short flight, in Alaska terms, to Fairbanks. As decoration, the airport in Fairbanks has stuffed Arctic animals in glass containers. Most New York museums would be envious of the collection. Everything from polar bears to eagles graced the wide corridors. The adventurers were mesmerized by the bears. Elroy stared at their sharp, white teeth and wondered how many smaller animals had been ripped and torn by them. Bears frightened him. Two taxis transported the adventurers to the Great Alaskan Hotel for needed sleep. The boys shared a room and the girls bunked together. Exhausted, they slept for nearly ten hours.

The next morning, they returned to the Fairbanks airport and met with the bush pilot that would ferry them to the cabin. His airplane would seat six, and it was decided that Janet and Anastasia would fly first to the wilderness cabin, along with some of the provisions. They would have roughly two hours to ready it before the next flight arrived consisting of Rusty, Trevor, Nicole, and Elroy. Ben would follow on the final flight, along with the rest of the supplies. It would take most of the day for the party and provisions to be transported to the cabin.

The bush pilot was obviously uncomfortable around physically and mentally impaired people. He was polite enough. He greeted us with a broad smile and shook our hands, except Rusty's. When he talked to everyone except Janet, he spoke slowly and loudly. He was in his early forties, short, and stocky. It appeared that flying had caused premature aging because his hair was almost completely gray. He sported a gray moustache and expensive pilot's sunglasses. He wore a baseball-type cap that had "Winslow Ground Service" printed on it. The single-engine airplane, obviously his pride and joy, was bright yellow. He loaded some of the supplies in the backseat and inside luggage compartment and other smaller boxes and duffel bags in an outside cranny. He explained to Janet that the airplane had to be balanced or takeoff would be compromised. After loading was done, he helped Anastasia in the back seat and fastened her seat and shoulder belts. Then, he helped Janet into the front passenger seat and carefully snapped the seat and shoulder belts. I felt like clubbing him with one of my metal canes.

I knew Janet must be the most attractive woman he had ever secured in that yellow airplane. I could tell he was awestruck with her beauty and manner, and he put on quite a show, strutting for her benefit. Flyboy was hitting on her, "Oh, look at me. I can fly an airplane." I've seen it all before, but it's still hard to deal with. I'm standing there with canes and spastic speech muscles, while the devil-may-care Flyboy is preparing to make my woman soar. Oh, it's sexual all right. Jealousy saturated my thoughts and I nearly panicked. What if Janet finally reached her senses and fell hopelessly in love with Flyboy, moved permanently to Alaska, never visited a pharmacy, and had twelve little Flyboys all sporting expensive sunglasses? I would be dumped by the only love of my pathetic, cerebral palsied life. I finally cooled down and realized that my insecurities were rearing their ugly heads. My brain again controlled my emotions. Love is blind faith, and I had to believe that Janet would remain mine. I had to believe that she saw through my rivals and never gave them a second thought. I had to believe that Janet was real and not some female aberration. I had to believe Janet had a blind spot. I waved to them as the airplane sped past us and slowly climbed into the great Alaskan sky. We walked back to the small coffee shop and awaited Flyboy's return.

Chapter Fifteen

The female grizzly bear had only been awake from her hibernation coma a few weeks. During the cold winter months, she had given birth to two cubs. They were constantly hungry and full of energy. After leaving the small cave, they began to descend the mountain, looking for food. The playful cubs frolicked and tumbled down hill after hill while the female grizzly searched for food. They finally reached a small tributary of the Dolores River and feasted on fish. The female grizzly began the task of teaching the cubs how to hunt and fare for themselves. The huge bear would spring onto her back legs and thrust her nose into the air, sniffing for prey. The cubs would imitate the behavior but tumble over. Early one evening, she detected a vaguely familiar smell, one she had experienced years ago at the William's City Dump. It was the scent of a human.

Chapter Sixteen

Janet hoped she wouldn't need the milk carton. Apparently, in smaller airplanes milk cartons served as barf bags. Her pilot said they also served as urinals on long flights when landing for a pit stop was out of the question. So far, so good, she thought. Her stomach and bladder were willing to contain their contents, at least for the moment. Besides, she doubted she could hit the container given the bumpy ride. The small airplane, and this one appeared to be the smallest of the small, bounced around like an old jalopy on a rocky road. She also thought this plane needed a muffler or something. One would certainly go deaf without the headset muffling the noise. She looked behind her and saw Anastasia with terror on her face. She reached for her hand, but it was pulled away. Anastasia did not want to be comforted.

The pilot had a big grin on his face as he made the necessary adjustment to keep the airplane aloft. He kept talking above the noise, shouting information about destination, speed, and scenic landmarks. Janet looked down at the miles of forest, rivers, mountains, and valleys and thought how beautiful Alaska was. Below, a herd of elk or reindeer ran across a river, frightened by the sound of the noisy airplane. Janet tried to signal Anastasia to the wild beauty below, but her eyes were closed tightly and she was muttering something to herself. When the pilot saw the stampeding herd, he banked the airplane sharply, lowered the nose, and shot over the herd, further scattering them. Flyboy called the maneuver a "buzz." It was a thrilling, beautiful sight.

Toward the end of the flight, Anastasia became more relaxed and even opened her eyes to the beauty below them. The rustic, log cabin approached in the distance. It was larger than Janet expected and nestled in a grove of trees just above the Dolores River. There was a small dirt landing strip about two football fields from it, where the airplane would land. Flyboy said he often used water pontoons in Alaska. Lakes and rivers provided ready-made smooth landing strips. But there was no lake close to the cabin, and the Dolores River was too shallow for a water landing. The yellow airplane banked and smoothly landed on the small dirt airstrip. After the propeller had ceased turning, Flyboy helped Janet and Anastasia out, and they walked the short distance to the two-story cabin. A fire was started in the old wood stove, and soon the cabin was warm and toasty. It was a beautiful retreat with golden wood floors, couches made of logs and cushions, and large windows overlooking the river. Anastasia was captivated by the large head of a long deceased moose overlooking the dining room. Janet and Anastasia began unpacking the supplies while they waited for grinning Flyboy and more adventurers.

Elroy was frightened and it was an overwhelming fear. The only reprieve he had from it was when he thought of Janet. Never did he entertain the thought that she was not leading a rescue in his direction, soon to embrace him with those wonderful, warm arms. Elroy was cold and shivering, and he looked around for warmth. He decided to crawl under a downed tree and hide from the cold and hungry bears. He kept thinking of the huge white teeth on the glass-enclosed airport bears. Twice, he shouted "Janet, I'm here." "Janet, I'm here."

In the distance, Ben saw Flyboy and his yellow airplane approach the airport. First, it was just a dot on the horizon and then a larger blot and finally a yellow blip with wings. After he landed and taxied to the flight center, Flyboy helped Elroy, Rusty, Nicole, and Trevor into the small airplane. Ben watched as they taxied to the end of the runway. He heard the engine rev, testing its strength, and then gradually gain speed until the three wheels lifted off the runway and into the Alaskan blue. He saw Nicole wave at him as the airplane dipped its wing and flew southwest toward the cabin. Ben plopped and slid back to the coffee shop to await his turn.

Janet and Anastasia waited patiently for the return of Flyboy and the rest of the crew. The two-hour wait turned into four and then six alarming hours. Patience turned to panic when a helicopter landed on the bank of the Dolores River, and Ben, the pilot, and a sheriff's deputy hurried to the cabin. The bad news was confirmed by the deputy, but he assured her that all that could be done was being done to find them.

They waited anxiously during the night. Early that morning, they heard the chop, chop, chop of the helicopter and saw it land. Elation turned to angst when all disembarked but Elroy. The pilot gave little hope of finding him. Alaska can be a desolate place. Air Search and Rescue frantically continued to scan the endless wilderness for Elroy or, God forbid, his body. Five airplanes, two helicopters, and three ground teams scoured a radius of fifty miles around the bobbing yellow airplane. The intense search continued for almost a week. On the sixth day, the deputy said they were going to call off the search for Elroy. They had given up hope. The weather or animals certainly had ended Elroy's life.

Chapter Seventeen

The world seems more frightening for people with high I.Q.s. Perhaps it is because they can imagine the multitude of things that can go wrong. When the word "ignorance" is used to signify low intelligence, then bliss can go hand-in-hand. Certainly, Elroy didn't feel bliss but he also didn't appreciate the gravity of his predicament. On the first day, he ran or walked over twenty miles from the crash scene. His bright red jacket would have been seen from the air had he not hidden under the dead tree. He slept there that night. On the second day, Elroy keep moving. He walked, rested, ran, rested, walked, and took shelter from the light rain under another downed tree. He was tired, hungry, and thirsty. He saw several bushes with green spring berries, but he never thought of them as edible. This was fortunate because they were poisonous. Throughout his ordeal, he had one and only one persistent thought: find Janet.

The news that the search was being discontinued caused Janet to cry and Ben to be outraged. But the Sheriff's deputy explained in logical detail that Elroy could be anywhere in a fifty square mile area. The rescuers felt it was likely that he had already fallen prey to wild animals or died from exposure. They said they had done all that could be done and expressed their heartfelt sorrow at their loss. After they left, Ben and Janet sat solemnly at the large wooden dinner table under the watchful dead eyes of the long-deceased moose and talked of options. After a few minutes, they both agreed that continuing the search for Elroy was the only acceptable one. They called the bush pilot who had spotted the wreck and hired him to continue the search. He would charge $175.00 per hour for each of the twelve hours of search time per day. Out of their sparse savings, Ben and Janet would pay nearly two thousand dollars per day to continue the search for Elroy. When that ran out, Ben would pay the pilot from his pension. He would quit the university, draw his pension in total, pay hefty taxes and penalties, and continue the search for Elroy until it too ran out. After their money ran out, Ben and Janet agreed they would search on foot. Never did they entertain the idea of quitting. They would give up the search for Elroy when he was found.

Several times, the female grizzly stood on her hind legs, sniffing the air. She definitely registered the scent of a human and began the search for her prey. The wind carried the scent, and she walked rapidly in the direction of its origin. The young cubs barely could keep up. She growled a hungry warning to other animals stalking the same prey. The female grizzly was no stranger to the hunt.

On the third day of the private search, Janet told Nyle to fly to the highest peak in the search radius. Trying to put herself in Elroy's place and knowing how he thought, it occurred to her that he would go to the highest peak. Elroy was like that. He would seek the brightest and highest. His optimism would dictate his course, and Janet wondered why she had not thought of it before. Nyle said the highest peak was nearly one hundred miles from the crash scene and he doubted Elroy or anyone could have traveled that far in such a short time. But he reluctantly agreed, and soon they were searching an 8,000-foot mountain peak with an idyllic lake nestled just below the summit.

Elroy reached the lake and drank icy cold water. He scooped the water into his hand and took gulp after gulp until satisfied. Muddy, he slid onto his side and, in a fetal position, began shaking from cold and fear. Overhead, he could hear the sound of an airplane, but he was too tired to wave or shout. In the trees bordering the lake, he heard a low-pitched growl and bushes rustling, but he was too tired to run, too tired to respond. He lay there dreaming of Janet, warmth, food, and the Center.

As the small airplane flew over the lake, Janet scanned the shoreline. At first, it appeared it was simply a rock of a different color, but as she stared at it, she thought she detected movement. She pointed to it and Nyle dipped the airplane wing to provide a better view. Then, she saw more movement and knew it was Elroy. Elation turned to terror when she saw a bear running from the trees toward him.

Chapter Eighteen

I hate funerals. They make me sad and they make me wonder. Unfortunately, I've attended more than my share of them. This funeral was basically the same as all of the others. I suppose that is the purpose of funerals, to be the same and to take thinking out of the process of bidding permanent farewell. Fortunately, I was spared the awful viewing of the body, because this one was closed casket. I hate plop, sliding by a dead person, gazing at the body, and wondering where the spark of life had gone. I think of dead bodies as shells; containers of thought and emotion. I wonder why people call them morticians rather than the more descriptive "undertakers." I wonder if my metal canes will be buried with me when I die?

Janet sat next to me while the speaker spoke of a life well-spent and of an untimely passing. If the quality of one's life is measured by how many people attend the funeral, then this life was well spent. The funeral was attended by hundreds of people, and many stood throughout the ritual at the back of the room. Relatives and friends spoke of family and friendship. Bitter and sweet memories were shared with all in attendance. Janet put her hand on mine as a song of remembrance was sung. Then, Elroy reached over, removed her hand from mine, and placed it firmly back in her lap. He's a cocky one, all right. When the song ended, we drove in the procession to Flyboy's final resting place. As the casket was lowered into the Alaskan ground, I wondered about life and death. Why do some people die from lost blood and other live because the sound of an airplane buzzing overhead frightens even the most determined of bears?

Chapter Nineteen

Steinbeck's *Of Mice and Men* disturbs me. It's not that Steinbeck isn't a great writer; the story disturbs me. So does the movie *Sling Blade*. They are both about murder and the mentally deficient. Ever since Bad Ron tried to kill Janet, I have been thinking about mentally deficient people and their capability for extreme good and evil. Just like the rest of us, they seem to possess tremendous good and devastating evil. In *Of Mice and Men*, Lennie Small kills because he doesn't understand his own strength. Karl Childers, in *Sling Blade*, kills because in his mind there are no other options. What motive did Bad Ron have for attempting to take my love from me? Was it out of frustration, lack of options, or simply brain chemistry gone awry? Bad Ron is back at the Center. He is watched by staff 24-7 and wears a chemical straightjacket. He is so medicated that violence is not an option.

What causes nobility in the mentally deficient? Where do the Elroy's of the world come from? Does loyalty, love, and courage spring from brain chemistry gone virtuous? Or, like in the rest of us, does it arise from the innate and unblocked goodness of humanity? Perhaps goodness cannot be suppressed by the lack of synapses and cortical sugar. As I scan the bright faces of my students desperately trying to relate to mice, men, California of the 1930s, and the reasons why the Pulitzer family awarded Steinbeck literary honor, I know that people and motives really never change. Humans, whether they are searching for a dream ranch or simply trying to survive the desperation of an economic and spiritual depression, are capable of nobility and ignominy. Intelligence is not the variable. It is all about heart, not mind.

Nearly six months have passed since our great Alaskan adventure. In my classroom, I see that the Bohemian has decided to weather yet another semester of the intellectually inferior waxing on and on about the rightness of their view. Apparently, she will tolerate discomfort in college and maybe learn something new, if not about them, then perhaps about herself. As I bring an end to my thoughts of mice and men, I bid the class a good homecoming. This weekend our football team will challenge the fighting team from another Midwestern university. It will be a gladiators' duel of honor for the benefit of those who have come home for the weekend.

Football Saturday is a grand time. I get up early and complete necessary Saturday "Honeydew" tasks, "Honey do this. Honey do that." I've lived in this small apartment for seven years, and I will miss it. Janet and I have started to search suburbia for our first home. Our realtor has called us several times with leads of fixeruppers that have just come on the market. He says now is a good time to buy as interest rates are probably going lower. But I'll miss this dump and the memories. I've grown comfortable here.

Janet's usual flat belly is bulging with signs of new life. I like it. In public places, I have the urge to point to my doings. After all, I sparked the growth all by myself and without the benefit of my canes. I did good. Poor Janet is buying ridiculous maternity clothing. She carries the baby well and looks great, but her body is expanding, her face is full, and she is beginning to waddle when she walks. Walking together, we must look quite the sight, waddle and plop-slide. Her regime of jogging has become a fast waddle-walk of half the distance.

Our marriage ceremony was small and intimate. It was held in the park at the Center, and nature kept the rain clouds away for most of it. There were about fifty people present and only one seizure. The chairs were aligned perfectly by several of the Center's residents, and the Park was adorned with flowers and streamers. It was a standard marriage. Janet wanted us to read our own prepared vows, but I was able to talk her out of it. Anxiety really tightens my spastic speech muscles. I can utter a simple "I do" clearly and articulately even when I'm panicked. But I was afraid that if I anxiously read a long list of promises and adornments, there would be mutterings in the audience: "Did he say he'd perish her for the rest of his wife?" "He has an infernal dove for her?" "What is that about his kart and troll?" Bob Charles was my best man, and when I asked for the ring, he searched his tuxedo in earnest. Or perhaps it was yet another example of British humor. I never can tell. Besides, we were both pretty hungover. I was surprised to find that Bob could throw a wicked bachelor's party. I was happy to discover that my singing prowess had not diminished over the years. Elroy and Trevor will never forget the stripper, and I'll never forget the sight of Rusty strobing while she performed. We all, in concert with Rusty, strobed while she gracefully removed her clothes to the bump and grind music. I wished I had a picture of that.

Elroy took the marriage well. Janet and I were concerned about how he'd react. But he sat in the front row with a smile on that big round face and seemed to enjoy it. I was afraid he'd object, jump to his feet and, in desperation, drag her down the aisle and away. But he simply sat, watched, and listened with that self-assured look on his face. Later, when the beautiful bride kissed him, he almost collapsed in euphoria. After the too long kiss, I shook his hand but he never lost eye-contact with Janet. As usual, I was just a nuisance and easily ignored. I had an urge to pull his hand forward, swing it above his head causing him to flip and sprawl prone on his back. He's a cocky little bugger.

Game time is 11:00 A.M. Janet and I plop-slide and waddle to the stadium along with the swelling mass of students and boosters. It is a beautiful fall morning. Hundreds of oak and maple trees show their colors. Football Saturday is a carnival and there is a magical crispness in the air. Today, there are jugglers and minstrels performing for pocket change, tail-gate parties of drunken football fans, and the blimp floating above it all. You can hear the echo of the marching band. We give our tickets to the guard and manage to find our seats on the second story of the stadium. I see that Bob has already arrived, and we greet each other. He offers us sips of his brandy-spiked hot chocolate and remarks that our team will again snatch defeat out of the jaws of victory. I suspect that because of the brandy he got the statement backwards, but then, with Bob, I really never know. Of course, alcoholic beverages are forbidden, but as tenured professors, we feel we have special privilege. Elroy and Janet share a sandwich as the coin is tossed. Our team elects to receive. We will accept the challenge.

The Silent Tongue (*aphasia*)

The words you do not hear the tears you cannot see
Are hidden within my nucleus, this is my new identity
I am alike dry earth, shriveled and worn
With no nurturing to the soul
And I am quite helpless, in my world no longer whole.
So bear with me and try to creep inside this silent tent
My ills have bereaved my spirit
My soul is discontent.

Please do not look at me . . . as if I am not here
Please do not speak to me . . . as if I cannot hear
Although I can't express myself with this muted speech of mine
My needs are very important it's difficult to define.
Please be polite and patient . . . maintain my dignity
My mind is tired and weary with this disability
I sit in silence in my room I cannot say "Good Morning Sun"
The words are tangled in my mind
Like twisted branches on a vine.

Those who speak in silence have a fervor
We . . . Who talk so freely don't understand or know
Take a walk into a garden, see the flowers row on row
Their colors are bright, their life is sweet
And we hear words of passion in the *silent way* they speak.

Kathleen Gerety, R.N.
Atkinson, New Hampshire
March 2002

SUGGESTED READING

Brumfitt, S. (1996). Losing your sense of self: What aphasia can do. In C. Code (ed.), *Forums in clinical aphasiology*, (pp. 349–355). London: Whurr Publishers.

Culbertson, W., Tanner, D., Peck, A., & Hooper, A. (1998). Orientation testing and responses of brain injured subjects. *Journal of Medical Speech-Language Pathology, 6*(2), 93–103.

Goldstein, K. (1952). The effects of brain damage on the personality. *Psychiatry, 15,* 245–260.

Huttlinger, K. & Tanner, D. (1994). The peyote way: Implications for culture care theory. *Journal of Transcultural Nursing, 5*(2), 5–11.

Keller, C., Tanner, D., Urbina, C., & Gerstenberger, D. (1989). Psychological responses in aphasia: Theoretical considerations and nursing implications. *Journal of Neuroscience Nursing, 21*(5), 290–294.

Rollin, W. (1987). *The psychology of communication disorders in individuals and their families.* Englewood Cliffs, NJ: Prentice-Hall.

Sarno, J. (1981). Emotional aspects of aphasia. In M. Sarno (ed.), *Acquired aphasia* (pp. 465–484). New York: Academic Press.

Tanner, D. & Gerstenberger, D. (1996). Clinical forum 9: The grief model in aphasia. In C. Code (ed.), *Forums in clinical aphasiology* (pp. 313–318). London: Whurr Publishers

Tanner, D. (1999). *The family guide to surviving stroke and communication disorders.* Boston: Allyn & Bacon.

Tanner, D. (1998). *Handbook for the speech-language pathology assistant.* Oceanside, CA: Academic Communication Associates.

Tanner, D. (1980). Loss and grief: Implications for the speech-language pathologist and audiologist. *ASHA, 22,* 916–928.

Weinstein, E., Lyerly, O., Cole, M., & Ozer, M. (1966). Meaning in jargon aphasia. *Cortex, 2,* 165–187.

Weinstein, E. & Puig-Antich, J. (1974). Jargon and its analogues. *Cortex, 10,* 75–83.

GLOSSARY

"Lexicographer: A writer of dictionaries, a harmless drudge."
—Samuel Johnson

The following books and dictionaries were consulted in selecting and defining some of the terms in this glossary:

Anderson, K. (ed.). (1998). *Mosbys medical, nursing & allied health dictionary*, (4th ed.). St. Louis, MO: Mosby.

Bear, M., Connors, B. & Paradiso, M. (1996). *Neuroscience: Exploring the brain*. Baltimore: Williams & Wilkins.

Boyd, M. & Nihart, M. (eds.) (1998). *Psychiatric nursing*. Philadelphia: Lippincott.

Culbertson, W. & Tanner, D. (1997). *Speech and hearing anatomy and physiology workbook*. Boston: Allyn & Bacon.

Dirckx, J. (ed.). (1997). *Stedman's concise medical dictionary for health professionals*, (3rd ed.). Baltimore, MD: Williams & Wilkins.

Kent, R. (1997). *The speech sciences*. San Diego, CA: Singular Publishing Group, Inc.

Nicolosi, L., Harryman, E., & Krescheck, K. (1996). *Terminology of communication disorders*, (4th ed.). Baltimore, MD: Williams & Wilkins.

Shames, G., Wiig, E. & Secord, W. (1998). *Human communication disorders: An introduction*, (5th ed.). Boston, MA: Allyn & Bacon.

Stuart, G. & Laraia, M. (eds.). (1998). *Principles and practice of psychiatric nursing*, (6th ed.). St. Louis: Mosby.

Tanner, D. (1999). *The family guide to surviving stroke and communication disorders*. Boston: Allyn & Bacon.

Zemlin, W. (1998). *Speech and hearing science*, (4th ed.). Boston: Allyn & Bacon.

A-: A prefix indicating the complete absence of function or ability.

Abstract attitude: Ability to symbolize and categorize verbal and nonverbal information; generalized ability to understand relationships.

Abulia: The inability to make decisions or to perform voluntary movements; chronic procrastination.

Acalculia: The inability to perform and understand simple mathematics due to neurological injury.

Acceptance: In grieving, the final stage in the process of accepting unwanted change; placing loss into a larger framework and being removed from emotional involvement.

Acquired aphasia: Loss of language occurring after birth as a result of disease or injury.

Addition: In speech articulation, a sound placed in a word where there should not be one.

Agnosia: The inability to recognize and appreciate the significance of sensory stimuli; usually specific to one modality of communication.

Agrammatism: Loss of the ability to understand and use the grammar of a language. The omission of grammatical units of language.

Agraphia: The inability to write, secondary to central language deficits and not due to limb paralysis. The inability to express oneself in writing.

Alexia: The inability to read, not due to visual acuity deficits or blindness.

Altruism: Demonstration of concern for others.

Amnesia: Partial or complete inability to recognize or recall past events; loss of memory.

Amusia: Inability to create, produce, or comprehend musical sounds.

Aneurysm: A ballooning or swelling in a wall of an artery.

Anomia: Loss of the ability to recall words, not limited to nouns.

Anosognosia: The inability to perceive, recognize, and accept body parts; denial of disability.

Anoxia: Lack of oxygen to the brain.

Anterograde amnesia: Loss of the ability to form, store, and recall new memories.

Anxiety: Worry, angst, fear, and apprehension. Lacking a sense of well-being, or in the extreme, a feeling of impending doom.

Aphasia: Multimodality inability to encode, decode and/or manipulate symbols for the purposes of verbal thought and/or communication. The loss of language due to damage of the speech and language centers of the brain.

Aphonia: Loss of the ability to vibrate the vocal cords to produce voice. The complete lack of phonation; without voice.

Apoplexy: Cerebral vascular accident; a stroke.

Apraxia of speech: Loss of the ability to conceptualize, plan, and sequence motor speech due to a neurological disorder.

Aprosody: Loss of the rhythm and melody of speech.

Arousal: Increased awareness of and responsiveness to internal and external stimuli.

Articulation: Shaping compressed air from the lungs into individual speech sounds. The act of moving the vocal tract structures in such a manner that speech sounds are produced.

Aspiration: In phonetics, addition of the whispered glottal sound to the normal sound of a phoneme. In dysphagia, ingestion of food or liquid into the respiratory system.

Association: The internalization of information and the process of making it personally relevant; relating of experiences, perceptions, and thoughts.

Ataxic dysarthria: A subtype of dysarthria associated with damage to the cerebellum and the tracts leading to and from it.

Auditory-acoustic agnosia: Inability to perceive differences in speech and environmental signals. The inability to perceive salient auditory features.

Auditory closure: Process by which auditory stimuli are integrated into a perceptual whole.

Auditory discrimination: Ability to perceive differences in sounds.

Body image: Awareness of one's own body. A composite vision of oneself.

Breathy: Voice quality created by excessive leakage of air when the vocal cords vibrate.

Broca's area: The part of the brain largely responsible for expressive communication, located in the frontal lobe in the dominant cerebral hemisphere. The cortical area associated with expressive language and motor speech production.

Catastrophic reaction: In aphasia, a psychobiological breakdown resulting from excessive stimulation, frustration, and anxiety. A sudden overwhelming feeling of anxiety and the reaction to it.

Cerebral vascular accident (CVA): A disruption of the flow of blood to the brain; a stroke.

Cerebral dominance: Tendency for one cerebral hemisphere to be dominant over the other for a particular function.

Circumlocution: The substitution of a word to avoid a feared one; rearranging or rephrasing the original thought.

Using a substitute word for the one that cannot be remembered or spoken.

Closed-head injury (CHI): Cerebral trauma of the nonpenetrating type.

Coarticulation: Overlapping articulatory influences during connected speech.

Cognition: Mental functions that include reasoning and higher order information processing. The mental processes of thinking and judgment.

Compulsivity: Unwanted, recurring urges to perform an act.

Confabulation: Giving answers to questions with no regard for their truthfulness; making up false stories.

Connotation: In addition to what the word denotes, the affective and evaluative associations made by the speaker or listener.

Consciousness: Awareness of the self and the environment.

Consummation of communication: The satisfactory completion of a speech act.

Content words: Words that carry the most meaning, such as nouns and verbs.

Conversion deafness: Deafness resulting from psychic trauma; psychogenic deafness.

Conversion aphonia: Loss of voice resulting from psychic trauma; psychogenic aphonia.

Conversion: Somatization of an emotional conflict and the resulting disorder.

Coping styles: Habitual methods of adjusting to anxiety, stress, and unwanted changes.

Coprolalia: Unprovoked use of obscene or profane language; excessive swearing.

Decode: The process of breaking down and analyzing a signal, such as words and language, into its component parts.

Dementia: Generalized cognitive deterioration, including disorientation, impaired judgment, and memory defects; generalized intellectual deficits.

Denial: Refusal to perceive and recognize threatening, unpleasant, and intolerable realities.

Denotation: The objective referent for a word.

Depersonalization: The disruption and disintegration of one's self-concept.

Disorientation: Inaccurate judgments about time, place, person, and/or situation.

Displacement: Shift of emotion to a neutral or less-threatening person or object.

Dissociation: Separation and compartmentalizing of a person's consciousness or identity to minimize anxiety.

Distortion: In speech articulation, the indistinct production of a sound.

Dys-: A prefix indicating impaired, faulty, or deficient.

Dysarthrias: A group of neuromuscular speech disorders. Impaired speech due to neurological and/or muscular deficits.

Dysfluency: An interruption in the flow of speech marked by repetitions, prolongations, hesitations, or blocks. A breakdown in the rhythm of speech.

Dyskinesia: Abnormal voluntary movements.

Dystonia: Abnormal, involuntary rhythmic twisting of body structure.

Echolalia: The repetition of that which has recently been spoken. Automatically repeating or "parroting" something that has been heard.

Ego: One of the three aspects of the personality that is involved in evaluating, directing, and controlling actions in response to reality.

Ego weakness: Reduced strength of the aspect of the personality involved in evaluating, directing, and controlling actions in response to reality.

Ego restriction: Narrowing of self-involvement.

Egocentric: Self-centered.

Embolism: A mass obstructing a blood vessel that develops in one part of the vascular system and ends up in another.

Empathy: Recognizing and understanding the emotional state of another person.

Encode: The process of putting an idea or thought into a signal system such as speech and language.

Enunciate: To articulate speech sounds precisely.

Etiology: The cause of something.

Euphoria: Heightened sense of well-being.

Executive function: Cognitive skills involved in planning, organization, executing, and monitoring complex behaviors.

Expressive language: Use of conventional encoded symbols to communicate spoken, gestured, or written concepts. Expression of the speaker's psychological state.

Expressive aphasia: A neurologically based loss of the expressive components of speech and language: speaking, writing, and gesturing.

External frame of reference: The belief that life events are the result of chance, fate, or the actions of external or supernatural forces.

Extrapyramidal system: Cell nuclei and nerve fibers involved in automatic, unconscious aspects of motor coordination, posture, and movement; all of the descending pathways except those of the pyramidal system.

Facilitation: Enabling desired behaviors, reactions, and adjustments.

Fainting: Temporary loss of consciousness due to extreme psychological distress.

False negative: Test results indicating the absence of a pathology when, in fact, a pathology exists.

False positive: Test results indicating a pathology when, in fact, a pathology does not exist.

Fear: The expectation of unpleasantness.

Filler: An interruption in the flow of speech by sounds such as "uh," "um," and "er."

Flaccid dysarthria: Neuromuscular speech disorder associated with lower motor neuron damage.

Flaccid: A muscle that is relaxed and without tone. A weak or limp muscle.

Flat affect: Narrowed mood, emotions, and temperament; reduced subjective experience of emotion.

Fluent speech: Smooth and effortlessly produced speech without hesitations, interjections, or repetitions. The act of speaking smoothly and easily.

Function words: Word with a grammatical function; prepositions, articles, pronouns, conjunctions, etc. Words that are important grammatically.

Frame of reference: Beliefs, attitudes, and assumptions about the cause-effect of life events.

Functional communication: The ability to express and understand basic ideas, needs, and wants.

Gesture: Movement of the body to describe or reinforce communication.

Grapheme: Printed or written symbols.

Gray matter: Collection of neuronal cell bodies in the central nervous system. Gray-colored tissue of the brain and spinal cord, primarily made up of cell bodies.

Grief response: Predictable stages in the process of accepting unwanted change.

Gustatory agnosia: Disorder relating to the perception of taste.

Gustatory: Related to the sense of taste.

Guttural: Produced in the throat; pertaining to the throat or voice.

Harshness: Voice quality caused by excessive force of vocal cord vibration. Acoustic qualities associated with hypertension of the vocal folds.

Hemiparesis: Weakness of the muscles on one side of the body.

Hemiplegia: Paralysis of one half of the body.

Hemorrhage: Rupture and escape of blood from a vein or artery.

Hesitations: Unusually long pauses during speech.

Hippocampus: A structure located in the brain that plays a role in learning and memory.

Hoarseness: Raspy voice quality; combination of harsh and breathy voice qualities.

Homonymous hemianopsia: Defective vision in one half of the fields of both eyes. A disorder where the patient's visual field is limited to one half of his or her total visual world.

Hostility: Chronic antagonistic attitude or feeling.

Hyper-: Prefix meaning "too much."

Hyperkinesia: A disorder characterized by excessive uncontrolled movements.

Hypernasality: Excessive perceived nasality; too much nasal resonance.

Hypo-: Prefix meaning "too little."

Hypokinesia: Slow or diminished movements.

Hyponasality: Too little nasality on the nasal consonants; densality.

Hysterical aphonia: Loss of voice occurring because of psychogenic factors.

Hysterical deafness: Loss of hearing because of psychogenic factors.

Hysterical stuttering: Stuttering occurring because of psychogenic factors. Usually late onset stuttering often caused by extreme anxiety.

Id: One of the three aspects of the personality. The unconscious part of the psyche containing instinctual drives.

Ideational apraxia: Disruption of the ability to conceptualize and program a motor impulse.

Image: Mental representation of some aspect of reality.

Infarct: The sudden death of tissue because of a lack of blood supply.

Inspiration: During breathing, the process of taking air into the lungs.

Intellectualization: Excessive reasoning to avoid negative emotions. The use of reasoning to negate emotional stress.

Intelligence: The ability to reason, problem solve, acquire, and retain knowledge.

Intelligibility: The ability to be understood by a listener; usually measured as a percentage.

Internal monologue: Communicating with oneself; self-talk or inner speech.

Internal frame of reference: Belief that one can influence or control the outcome of events.

Ischemic: Inadequate flow of blood to a part of the body.

Jargon: Fluent but unintelligible speech; fluent speech that makes no sense.

Jargon aphasia: A type of aphasia where the patient utters fluent speech, but it makes little or no sense.

Kinesthesia: The perception of one's body movement. In speech, the perception of movement and direction of the speech musculature.

Language: The multimodality ability to encode, decode, and manipulate symbols for the purposes of verbal thought and/or communication. Rule-governed, socially shared code for representing concepts through the use of symbols.

Larynx: The voice box.

Limbic system: A group of interconnected structures involving emotion, memory, and learning.

Linguistic relativity: The concept that language affects thought.

Localization: In neurology, the identification of areas of the brain responsible for specific aspects of physical, mental, or emotional functioning.

Logorrhea: The continuous, fluent incoherent production of words.

Loudness: Psychological perception of amplitude or intensity of an acoustic signal.

Macroglossia: Abnormally large tongue relative to the oral cavity.

Mandible: The lower jaw.

Maxilla: The upper jaw.

Meninges: The three membranes surrounding the surface of the central nervous system; dura mater, arachnoid mater, and pia mater.

Metastasis: Migration and spreading of a disease from one location to another.

Microglossia: Abnormally small tongue relative to the oral cavity.

Mixed dysarthria: Two or more dysarthrias occurring concurrently or the changing of the dysarthria type over time.

Modality: Any avenue or mode of communication.

Morpheme: Smallest unit of meaning in language; minimum unit of speech that is meaningful.

Motor speech disorders: Pertaining to disorders of motor tracts and muscles; apraxia of speech and the dysarthrias.

Multiple personalities: Two or more distinct personalities within the same individual.

Mutism: Completely without speech; inability to phonate and articulate.

Nasal emission: Air released through the nose during speech; air flowing out of the nose.

Neologism: A made-up or invented word. A conventional word used in an unconventional manner.

Neuroscience: The interdisciplinary science that studies the brain, emotions, and behaviors.

Noise: Any signal that competes with the perception of a stimulus; unwanted sound.

Nonfluency: The absence of fluent speech.

Nonverbal communication: Communication without using spoken words.

Obsessive-compulsive: Persistent adherence to thoughts and beliefs and the need to perform certain rituals to excess.

Olfactory: Related to the sense of smell.

Olfactory agnosia: Disorder relating to the perception of odors.

Oral apraxia: Loss of the ability to conceptualize, plan, and sequence voluntary oral nonspeech movements due to a neurological disorder.

Orientation: Awareness of time, place, person, and situation.

Palsy: Paresis or paralysis of a muscle.

Paraphasia: Aphasic naming disorder characterized by choosing the incorrect word that either rhymes or has a semantic relationship to the correct one; literal and verbal paraphasias.

Perception: Realizing the significance of sensory information; awareness and appreciation of the salient aspects of a stimulus. Organization and interpretation of incoming sensory information.

Perseveration: The automatic continuation of a speaking or writing response seen in some patients with neurogenic communication disorders. Sensory and motor responses that persist for a longer duration than what would be warranted by the intensity and significance of the stimuli.

Phobia: Excessive and abnormal fear.

Phonation: Any voiced sound that occurs at the level of the vocal cords. Transformation of acoustic energy within the larynx by means of vocal fold vibration.

Phonatory apraxia: Loss of the ability to conceptualize, plan, and sequence voluntary laryngeal movements due to a neurological disorder.

Phonetics: The study of the acoustics, perception, classification, description, and production of speech sounds of a language.

Phonology: The study of the sounds of a language and the way they are combined into words. The study of the sound system of a language.

Pitch: Psychological perception of frequency of vibration.

Prognosis: A prediction about how well a patient will recover from a disease, disorder, or disability.

Projection: Attributing one's own intolerable wishes, thoughts, motivations, and feelings to another person.

Propositionality: The meaningfulness and amount of content in an utterance.

Prosody: Patterns of speech such as stress, intonation, rhythm, melody, and pitch.

Psychoacoustics: Study of psychological responses to sound.

Psychogenic: Of emotional or affective origin.

Psychology: The study of human consciousness. Methods of measuring, explaining, and changing behavior in humans and other animals.

Quadriplegia: Paralysis or weakness of all four extremities.

Quality: In voice, the perceptual correlate of complexity of acoustic signals; the spectral characteristics of a sound.

Quality of life: Combination of factors that contribute to satisfaction with life.

Rate of speech: The speed of speaking usually measured in words per minute.

Rationalization: The attempt to justify or make acceptable intolerable feelings, behaviors, and motives.

Reaction formation: Avoidance of anxiety by engaging in thoughts and behaviors that are opposite of what one would really like to do.

Receptive aphasia: A neurologically based loss of the receptive components of language: auditory comprehension, reading, gesturing.

Receptive language: The use of conventional decoded symbols to understand phonemes, words, gestures, and graphemes.

Referent: The aspect of reality referred to by the symbol.

Regression: In psychology, the retreat to an earlier and more comfortable level of development and adjustment, due to stress.

Rehabilitation: Therapeutic restoration of a deficient function, such as communication, to normal or near-normal levels.

Reinforcement: The positive or negative consequences of a behavior.

Repression: Involuntary exclusion of a painful thought or memory from awareness.

Respiration: The act of breathing; inspiration and expiration.

Retrograde amnesia: Amnesia of events prior to an illness or traumatic injury to the brain.

Screening: A gross measurement of a function to determine the need for additional testing; testing to detect the presence of a disorder.

Seizure: A spontaneous excessive discharge of cortical neurons.

Self-concept: Awareness of oneself particularly in relation to others; images and definitions of self.

Self-esteem: Positive belief and feelings about one's self-concept.

Semantics: The meaning of words. The relationship between a symbol and what it represents.

Senility: Cognitive and intellectual deterioration associated with pathological aging.

Short-term memory: Temporary storage of information requiring continual rehearsal.

Soft palate: The soft muscular part located at the back of the roof of the mouth. The muscle at the back of the hard palate; the velum.

Sound discrimination: The auditory ability to perceive the difference between two sounds, especially similar ones.

Spasm: An involuntary contraction of a muscle or a muscle group.

Spastic: A form of paralysis where a muscle is contracted all of the time due to a neurological injury or disease; hypertonicity.

Spastic dysarthria: Neuromuscular speech disorder associated with bilateral upper motor lesions.

Speech act: The verbal expression of an intent; an act of propositional verbal communication.

Split-brain studies: Studies of brain functioning following the disconnection of all or part of the corpus callosum.

Spontaneous recovery: The period of time post onset where the brain naturally resolves part or all of the neurogenic disorder.

Stress: Mental and emotional tension arising from fear, anxiety, conflicts, temporal urgency, and excessive stimulation.

Stroke: A sudden deprivation of the blood supply to the brain; cerebral vascular accident.

Subcortical: The areas of the brain below the cerebral cortex.

Sublimation: Engaging in a socially acceptable substitute pattern of behavior for one that is blocked in an effort to reduce anxiety.

Superego: One of the three aspects of the personality that is involved with values, ethics, and conscience.

Suppression: Intentional exclusion of thoughts and feelings from consciousness.

Syndrome: A combination or cluster of symptoms that usually occur together.

Syntax: The grammatical structure of language, especially word order.

Tachylalia: Excessive rate of speech.

Tactile: Relating to the sense of touch.

Tactile agnosia: Disorder relating to the perception of touch.

Transient ischemic attack (TIA): Like a stroke, but does not result in permanent damage to the brain and lasts fewer than twenty-four hours.

Telegraphic speech: Communication using a minimum of function words and using a high number of content words, similar to a telegram.

Tempo: The rate or speed of speaking.

Thorax: The chest.

Tremor: Oscillation or vibration of a muscle or structure of the body.

Tic: A sudden twitch; an involuntary repeated contraction of a muscle or muscle group.

Trachea: The windpipe.

Tract: Central nervous system axons having a common origin and destination; anatomically related parts of the central nervous system.

Traumatic brain injury (TBI): Injury to the brain caused by a blunt force or a penetrating object.

Undoing: An act or communication that attempts to reverse or negate a previous one.

Unilateral neglect: Difficulty attending to one side of the body.

Velopharyngeal closure: The closing off of the nasal cavity by the actions of the velum and pharynx.

Velum: The soft palate.

Ventricles: Interconnected, fluid-filled cavities in the brain.

Visual agnosia: Disorder relating to the perception of written words, forms, and objects.

Visual neglect: Lack of attention to a particular space or visual field.

Wernicke's area: The part of the dominant hemisphere of the brain largely responsible for receptive language.

REFERENCES

Baker, M. & Tanner, D. (1990, April). *Recovery from brain insult: Investigation of patient and family adaptation.* Paper presented to the annual convention of the Canadian Association of Speech-Language Pathologists and Audiologists, Vancouver, BC.

Battista, J. (1982). Empirical test of Valiant's hierarchy of ego functions. *American Journal of Psychiatry, 139,* 356–357.

Benson, D. F. & Ardila, A. (1996). *Aphasia.* New York: Oxford University Press.

Benson, D. F. (1993). Aphasia. In K. Heilman & E. Valenstein (eds.), *Clinical neuropsychology* (pp. 17–36). New York: Oxford University Press.

Benton, A. (1981). Aphasia: Historical perspectives. In M. Sarno (ed.), *Acquired aphasia* (pp. 1–25). New York: Academic Press.

Black, F. (1975). Unilateral brain lesions and MMPI performance: A preliminary study. *Perceptual and Motor Skills, 40,* 87–93.

Boyd, M. (1998a). Theoretical basis of psychiatric nursing. In M. Boyd & M. Nihart (eds.), *Psychiatric nursing* (pp. 110–151). Philadelphia: Lippincott.

Boyd, M. (1998b). Biopsychosocial aspects of stress and crisis. In M. Boyd & M. Nihart (eds.), *Psychiatric nursing* (pp. 296–336). Philadelphia: Lippincott.

Brain, R. (1965). Speech disorders: Aphasia, apraxia and agnosia, (2nd ed.). Washington, DC: Butterworth.

Bridge, C. & Twible, R. (1997). Clinical reasoning: Informed decision making for practice. In C. Christiansen & C. Baum (eds.) *Occupational therapy* (2nd ed.) Thorofare, NJ: Slack, Incorporated.

Brumfitt, S. (1996). Losing your sense of self: What aphasia can do. In C. Code (ed.) *Forums in clinical aphasiology* (pp. 349–369). London: Whurr Publishers.

Burgess, A. & Clements, P. (1998). Stress, coping, and defensive functioning. In A. Burgess (ed.), *Psychiatric nursing* (pp. 77–90). Stamford, CT: Appleton & Lange.

Carlat, D. (1999). *The psychiatric interview.* Philadelphia: Lippincott, Williams & Wilkins.

Carson, R., Butcher, J., & Coleman, J. (1988). *Abnormal psychology and modern life.* Glenview, IL: Foresman and Company.

Chapman, A. (1976). *Textbook of clinical psychiatry,* (2nd ed.). Philadelphia: Lippincott.

Chisholm, M. (1993). Anxiety. In R. Rawlins, S. Williams & C. Beck (eds.), *Mental health-psychiatric nursing* (3rd ed.). St. Louis: Mosby.

Craig, A. & Cummings, J. (1995). Neuropsychiatric aspects of aphasia. In H. Kirshner (ed.), *Handbook of neurological speech and language disorders* (pp. 483–498). New York: Marcel Dekker, Inc.

Critchley, M. (1970). *Aphasiology and other aspects of language.* London, UK: Edward Arnold.

Crowe, T. (1997). Theories of personality. In T. Crowe (ed.), *Applications of counseling in speech-language pathology and audiology* (pp. 48–79). Baltimore: Williams & Wilkins.

Culbertson, W., Tanner, D., Peck, A., & Hooper, A. (1998). Orientation testing and responses of brain injured subjects. *Journal of Medical Speech-Language Pathology, 6*(2), 93–103.

Damico, J.S., Oelschlaeger, M., & Simmons-Mackie, N.N. (1999). Qualitative methods in aphasia research: conversation analysis. *Aphasiology, 13,* 667–680.

Darley, F., Aronson, A., & Brown, J. (1975). *Motor speech disorders.* Philadelphia: Saunders.

Darley, F. (1982). *Aphasia.* Philadelphia: Saunders.

DeGroef, J. & Heinemann, E. (1999). *Psychoanalysis and mental handicap.* London: Free Association Books.

181

Duchan, J.F. (2000). Preface from situating language assessment: Influences from the past, directions for the future. *Seminars in Speech and Language, 21,* 189–192.

Duffy, J. (1995). *Motor speech disorders.* St. Louis: Mosby.

Eisenson, J. (1984). *Adult aphasia,* (2nd ed.). Englewood Cliffs, NJ: Prentice-Hall.

Fitzhenry, R. (1993). *The Harper book of quotations* (3rd ed.). New York: Harper-Perennial.

Frank, C. (1998). Overview of psychiatric disease for the speech-language practitioner. In A. Johnson & B. Jacobson (eds.), *Medical speech-language pathology: A practitioner's guide* (pp. 637–654). New York: Thieme.

Freud, S. (1908). *Character and anal erotism.* (Standard ed., Vol. 9). London, UK: Hogarth Press.

Gainotti, G. (1972). Emotional behavior and hemisphere side of the lesion. *Cortex, 8,* 41–55.

Gainotti, G. (1989). The meaning of emotional disturbances resulting from unilateral brain injury. In G. Gainotti & C. Caltagirone (eds.), *Emotions and the dual brain* (pp. 147–167). New York: Springer-Verlag.

Gasparini, W., Satz, P., Heilman, K., & Coolidge, F. (1978). Hemispheric asymmetries of affective processing as determined by the Minnesota multiphasic personality inventory. *Journal of Neurology, Neurosurgery and Psychiatry, 41,* 470–473.

George, K., Vikingstad, E., & Cao, Y. (1998). Brain imaging in neurocommunicative disorders. In A. Johnson & B. Jacobson (eds.), *Medical speech-language pathology: A practitioner's guide* (pp. 285–336), New York: Thieme.

Geschwind, N. (1967). The varieties of naming errors. *Cortex.* 3(1), 97–112.

Gillis, R. (1996). *Traumatic brain injury rehabilitation for speech-language pathologists.* Boston: Butterworth-Heinemann.

Goldstein, K. (1924). Das wesen der amnestischen aphasia. *Schweizer Archiv fuer Neurologia and Psychiatrie, 15,* 163–175.

Goldstein, K. (1948). *Language and language disturbances.* New York: Grune and Stratton.

Goldstein, K. (1952). The effects of brain damage on the personality. *Psychiatry, 15,* 245–260.

Goldstein, K. (1959). Functional disturbances in the brain. In S. Arieti (ed.), *American handbook of psychiatry.* New York: Basic Books.

Gordon, W., Hibbard, M., Egelko, S., & Diller, L. (1985). The multifaceted nature of the cognitive deficits following stroke: Unexpected findings. *Archives of Physical Medicine and Rehabilitation, 66,* 338.

Gordon, W., Hibbard, M., & Morganstein, S. (1996). Response to Tanner and Gerstenberger. In C. Code (ed.), *Forums in clinical aphasiology* (pp. 319–321). London, UK: Whurr Publishers.

Heilman, K., Bowers, D., & Valenstein, E. (1993). Emotional disorders associated with neurological diseases. In K. Heilman & E. Valenstein (eds.), *Clinical neuropsychology* (pp. 461–498). New York: Oxford University Press.

Heilman, K. & Valenstein, E. (1993). Introduction. In K. Heilman, and E. Valenstein (eds.), *Clinical neuropsychology* (pp. 3–16). New York: Oxford University Press.

Herrmann, M., Barrels, C., & Wallesch, C. (1993). Depression in acute and chronic aphasia: Symptoms, pathoanatomical-clinical correlations and functional implications. *Journal of Neurology, Neurosurgery, and Psychiatry, 56*(6), 672–678.

Herrmann, M. & Wallesch, C. (1989). Psychosocial changes and psychosocial adjustments with chronic and severe non-fluent aphasia. *Aphasiology, 3*(6), 513–526.

Holland, A. & Beeson, P. (1995). Aphasia therapy. In H. Kirshner (ed.), *Handbook of neurological speech and language disorders* (pp. 445–464). New York: Marcel Dekker, Inc.

Huelskoetter, M. (1983). The person who uses dysfunctional coping patterns. In C. Beck, R. Rawlins, & S. Williams (eds.), *Mental health-psychiatric nursing.* St. Louis: Mosby.

Huttlinger, K. & Tanner, D. (1994). The peyote way: Implications for culture care theory. *Journal of Transcultural Nursing, 5*(2), 5–11.

Imboden, J. & Urbaitis, J. (1978). *Practical psychiatry in medicine.* New York: Appleton-Century-Crofts.

Jacobson, A., Beardslee, W., & Hauser, S. (1986a). An approach to evaluating ego defense mechanisms using clinical interviews. In G. Valiant (ed.), *Empirical studies of the ego mechanisms of defense.* Washington, DC: American Psychiatric Press.

Jacobson, A., Beardslee, W., & Hauser, S. (1986b). Evaluating ego defense mechanisms using clinical interviews: An empirical study of adolescent diabetic and psychiatric patients. *Journal of Adolescence, 9,* 303–319.

Keller, C., Tanner, D., Urbina, C., & Gerstenberger, D. (1989). Psychological responses in aphasia: Theoretical considerations and nursing implications. *Journal of Neuroscience Nursing, 21*(5), 290–294.

Kolb, L. (1977). *Modern clinical psychiatry.* Philadelphia: Saunders.

Kübler-Ross, E. (1969). *On death and dying.* New York: Macmillan.

LaPointe, L. & Katz, R. (1998). Neurogenic disorders of speech. In G. Shames, E. Wiig, & W. Secord (eds.), *Human communication disorders* (5th ed.) (pp. 434–471). Boston: Allyn & Bacon.

LaPointe, L. (1997). Adaptation, accommodation, aristos. In L. LaPointe (ed.), *Aphasia and related neurogenic language disorders* (2nd ed.). New York: Thieme.

Laraia, M. (1998). Biological context of psychiatric nursing care. In G. Stuart & M. Laraia (eds.), *Principles and practice of psychiatric nursing* (6th ed.) (pp. 88–119). St. Louis: Mosby.

Larson, M. (1984). Flexibility-Rigidity. In C. Beck, R. Rawlins, & S. Williams (eds.), *Mental health-psychiatric nursing* (pp. 537–562). St. Louis: Mosby.

Lawton, M. (1991). A multidimensional view of quality of life in frail elders. In J. Birren (ed.), *The concept and measurement of quality of life in frail elders* (pp. 4–23). San Diego: Academic Press.

Lipsey, J., Spencer, W., Rabins, P., & Robinson, R. (1986). Phenomenological comparison of poststroke depression and functional depression. *American Journal of Psychiatry, 143,* 4.

Luria, A. (1958). Brain disorders and language analysis. *Language and Speech, 1,* 14–34.

Luria, A. (1964). Factors and forms of aphasia. In A. DeReuck & M. O'Connor (eds.), *Disorders of language.* London: J. & A. Churchill

Luria, A. (1966). *Higher cortical function in man.* New York: Basic Books.

Luria, A. (1970). *Traumatic aphasia: Its syndromes, psychology and treatment.* The Hague: Mouton.

Luria, A. (1974). Language and brain. *Brain and Language, 1,* 1–14.

MacNeil, B., Weischselbaum, R., & Pauker, S. (1981). Tradeoffs between quality and quality of life in laryngeal cancer. *New England Journal of Medicine, 305,* 983–987.

Mahl, G. (1971). *Psychological conflict and defense.* New York: Hartcourt Brace Jovanovich.

Marquardt, T. (2000). Acquired neurogenic language disorders. In R. Gillam, T. Marquardt, & F. Martin (eds.), *Communication sciences and disorders* (pp. 461–485). San Diego: Singular.

Oakley, L. (1998). Socioculture context of psychiatric nursing. In G. Stuart & M. Laraia (eds.), *Principles and practice of psychiatric nursing* (6th ed.). St. Louis: Mosby.

Owens, R., Metz, D., & Haas, A. (2000). *Introduction to communication disorders.* Boston: Allyn & Bacon.

Perry, J. & Cooper, S. (1986). A preliminary report on defenses and conflicts associated with borderline personality disorders. *Journal of American Psychology Association, 34,* 864–895.

Perry, J. & Cooper, S. (1987). Empirical studies of psychological defense mechanisms. In J. Cavenar (ed.), *Psychiatry - Volume I*, Philadelphia: Lippincott.

Prazich, M. (1985). *A stroke patient's own story*. Danville, IL: Interstate Printers and Publishers.

Ritchie, D. (1961). *Stroke: A study of recovery*. Garden City, NJ: Doubleday.

Robinson, R., & Benson, D. F. (1981). Depression in aphasic patients: Frequency, severity, and clinical-pathological correlations. *Brain and Language, 14*, 282–291.

Robinson, R., Boston, J., Starkstein, S. & Price, T. (1988). Comparison of mania and depression after brain injury: Causal factors. *American Journal of Psychiatry, 145*, 2.

Robinson, R., Lipsey, J., Bolla-Wilson, K, Bolduc, P., Pearlson, G, Rao, K., & Price, T. (1985). Mood disorders in left-handed stroke patients. *American Journal of Psychiatry 142*, 12.

Robinson, R. (1986). Depression and stroke. *Psychiatric Annals, 17*(11), 731–740.

Rollin, W. (1987). *The psychology of communication disorders in individuals and their families*. Englewood Cliffs, NJ: Prentice-Hall.

Ryalls, J. & Behrens, S. (2000). *Introduction to speech sciences*. Boston: Allyn & Bacon.

Sackeim, H., Greenberg, M., Weiman, A., Gur, R., Hungerbahler, J., & Geschwin, N. (1982). Hemispheric asymmetry in the expression of positive and negative emotions: Neurological evidence. *Archives of Neurology, 39*, 210–218.

Sackeim, H. & Weber, S. (1982). Functional brain asymmetry in the regulation of emotion: Implications for bodily manifestations of stress. In L. Goldberger & S. Breznitz (eds.), *Handbook of stress*. New York: Macmillan.

Sarason, I. & Sarason, B. (1993). *Abnormal Psychology: The problem of maladaptive behavior*. Englewood Cliffs, NJ: Prentice-Hall.

Sarno, M. (1991). Treatment of aphasia workshop research and research needs. *Aphasia treatment: Current approaches and research opportunities, 2*, 11–16.

Sarno, J. (1981). Emotional aspects of aphasia. In M. Sarno (ed.), *Acquired aphasia*

(pp. 465–484). New York: Academic Press.

Schuell, H., Jenkins, J., & Jimenez-Pabon, E. (1964). *Aphasia in adults*. New York: Harper and Row.

Scott, K. & Tanner, D. (1990, April). *Recovery from brain insult: Investigation of patient adaptation and recovery*. Paper presented to the annual convention of the Canadian Association of Speech-Language Pathologists and Audiologists, Vancouver, BC.

Sies, L. (1974). *Aphasia: Theory and therapy*. Baltimore: University Park Press.

Stuart, G. & Laraia, M. (1998). *Principles and practice of psychiatric nursing* (6th ed.). St. Louis: Mosby.

Stuart, G. (1998). Self-concept responses and dissociative disorders. In G. Stuart & M. Laraia (eds.), *Principles and practice of psychiatric nursing* (6th ed.). St. Louis: Mosby

Stuart, G. (2001a). Self-concept responses and dissociative disorders. In G. Stuart & M. Laraia (eds.), *Principles and practice of psychiatric nursing* (7th ed.) (pp. 317–344). St. Louis: Mosby.

Stuart, G. (2001b). Anxiety responses and anxiety disorders. In G. Stuart & M. Laraia (eds.), *Principles and practice of psychiatric nursing* (7th ed.) (pp. 274–298). St. Louis: Mosby.

Swindell, C., Holland, A. & Reinmuth, O. (1998). Aphasia and related adult disorders. In G. Shames, E. Wiig & W. Secord (eds.), *Human communication disorders* (pp. 472–509). Boston: Allyn & Bacon.

Tanner, D., Baker, M., Culbertson, W., & Palcich, W. (1993, November). *Adjustment and speech recovery in CVA and TBI patients*. Paper presented to the Annual Convention of the American Speech and Hearing Association, Anaheim, CA.

Tanner, D. & Barnwell, J. (1994). *The psychology of global aphasia: Theoretical and practical issues*. Miniseminar presented to the Annual Convention of the American-Speech-Language-Hearing Association, New Orleans, LA.

Tanner, D. & Gerstenberger, D. (1988). The grief response in neuropathologies of speech and language. *Aphasiology, 1*(6), 79–84.

Tanner, D. & Gerstenberger, D. (1989). *Psychological conflict and defense in aphasia.* Miniseminar presented at the Annual Convention of the American-Speech-Language-Hearing Association, St. Louis, MO.

Tanner, D. & Gerstenberger, D. (1996). Clinical forum 9: The grief model in aphasia. In C. Code (ed.), *Forums in clinical aphasiology* (pp. 313–318). London: Whurr Publishers

Tanner, D. & Huttlinger, K. (1989). *Peyote in the treatment of post traumatic aphasia: A case study.* Paper presented at the Annual Meeting of the American Society for Applied Anthropology, Santa Fe, NM.

Tanner, D. (1980). Loss and grief: Implications for the speech-language pathologist and audiologist. *ASHA, 22,* 916–928.

Tanner, D. (1987). *The family's guide to stroke, head trauma and speech disorders.* Tulsa, OK: Modern Education Corporation.

Tanner, D. (1996). *An introduction to the psychology of aphasia.* Dubuque, IA: Kendall-Hunt.

Tanner, D. (1997). *Aphasia: Coping with unwanted change* (Rev. Ed.) Dubuque, IA: Kendall-Hunt.

Tanner, D. (1999). *The family guide to surviving stroke and communication disorders.* Boston: Allyn & Bacon.

Tetnowski, J.A., & Damico, J.S. (2001). A demonstration of the advantages of qualitative methodologies in stuttering research. *Journal of Fluency Disorders, 26,* 17–42.

Trousseau, A. (1865). *Clinique medicale de l'Hotel-Dieu de Paris* (2nd ed.). Paris: J.B. Bailliere.

Valiant, G. & Drake, R. (1985). Maturity of ego defenses in relation to DSM-III Axis II personality disorder. *Archives of general psychiatry, 42,* 597–601.

Valiant, G. (1977). *Adaptation to life.* Boston: Little, Brown, and Co.

Van Riper, C. & Erickson, R. (1996). *Speech correction.* Boston: Allyn & Bacon.

Währborg, P. (1996). Aphasia and family therapy. In C. Code (ed.), *Forums in clinical aphasiology* (pp. 333–339). London: Whurr Publishers.

Walker, J. (1981). *Clinical psychiatry in primary care.* Menlo Park, CA.: Addison-Wesley.

Weinstein, E., Lyerly, O., Cole, M., & Ozer, M. (1966). Meaning in jargon aphasia. *Cortex, 2,* 165–187.

Weinstein, E. & Puig-Antich, J. (1974). Jargon and its analogues. *Cortex, 10,* 75–83.

Weisenburg, T. & McBride, K. (1935). *Aphasia.* New York: Commonwealth Fund. (Reprinted in 1964, New York: Hafner.).

Wepman, J., & Jones, L. (1961). *Studies in aphasia: An approach to testing.* Chicago: University of Chicago Press.

Wepman, J. & Jones, L. (1966). Speech, language and communication. In E. Carterette (ed.), *Brain function.* Los Angeles: University of California Press.

Wepman, J. (1962). The language disorders. In J. Garrett & E. Levine (eds.), *Psychological practices with the physically disabled* (pp. 197–230). New York: Columbia University Press.

Wolberg, R. (1977). *The technique of psychotherapy* (3rd ed.). New York: Grune and Stratton.

Zemlin, W. (1998). *Speech and hearing science* (4th ed.). Boston: Allyn & Bacon.

INDEX

Note: Page numbers for Figures or Tables are in *italics*.